Advance Praise for
The Energy Prescription

"*The Energy Prescription* integrates the best of alternative medicine with the mind-body traditions of indigenous wisdom. A practical manual for anyone who knows that our energy connection must be monitored and nurtured consciously."
—James Redfield, author of *The Celestine Prophecy*

"In *The Energy Prescription*, Connie Grauds shows how to get back on track to live a vital and fulfilling life. Taking wisdom from ancient shamanistic approaches, she shows how to heal such common and persistent problems as chronic fatigue, depression, and anxiety by helping us connect to the deepest parts of ourselves."
—Carol Adrienne, Ph.D., author of
When Life Changes, or You Wish It Would

"Connie Grauds has a most intriguing perspective on health and healing: trained as a pharmacist, she has spent years studying with a shaman in the Peruvian Amazon. As such, she offers interesting insights into treatments for problems like depression and insomnia, ailments that she terms 'energy leaks.' I recommend this book for anyone interested in holistic healing."
—Mark J. Plotkin, president, Amazon Conservation
Team, and author of *Tales of a Shaman's Apprentice*

The Energy Prescription

Give Yourself Abundant Vitality
with the Wisdom of
America's Leading Natural Pharmacist

CONNIE GRAUDS, R.Ph.
AND DOUG CHILDERS

Foreword by Larry Dossey, M.D.

BANTAM BOOKS

THE ENERGY PRESCRIPTION
A Bantam Book / August 2005

Published by
Bantam Dell
A Division of Random House, Inc.
New York, New York

Book design by Lynn Newmark

Bantam Books and the rooster colophon are registered trademarks of Random
House, Inc.

Library of Congress Cataloging-in-Publication Data
Grauds, Connie.
The energy prescription : give yourself abundant vitality with the wisdom of
America's leading natural pharmacist / Connie Grauds and Doug
Childers ; foreword by Larry Dossey.
p.   cm.
Includes bibliographical references and index.
ISBN 0-553-38254-3
1. Shamanism. 2. Health. 3. Vital force. 4. Naturopathy. I. Childers, Douglas.
II. Title.

RZ999.G697 2005
615.5'35—dc22
2005041019

Printed in the United States of America
Published simultaneously in Canada

www.bantamdell.com

BVG 10 9 8 7 6 5 4 3 2 1

CONTENTS

Section Three:
The Five Common Energy Leaks

Section Four:
Nature's Energy Medicine Chest

ACKNOWLEDGMENTS

A special note of thanks and appreciation to the following: don Antonio, Larry Dossey, Arielle Eckstut, Kitty Farmer, and Philip Rappaport.

A note of gratitude for their spirited contribution: Grace and Flo.

FOREWORD

I.

From the mountainside where I live in northern New Mexico, I gaze upon two different worlds. In the far distance I can see the glistening roofs of Los Alamos, the most famous weapons laboratory in the world, nestled against the Jemez Mountains. Here, during World War II, the Manhattan Project scientists created the atomic bombs that were dropped on the Japanese cities of Hiroshima and Nagasaki. And in the middle distance, only a few miles away, I see the valley of the Rio Grande, along which stand several ancient pueblos.

A more striking contrast in civilizations and worldviews can hardly be imagined. In the pueblos, life remains attuned to the rhythms of the land and river. Ideas such as harmony with nature and the sacredness of all things are still honored. Pueblo healers continue to believe that health requires attention to the soul, and that damage to or loss of the soul sets the stage for illness, ideas discussed in this fine book by Constance Grauds and Douglas Childers. At Los Alamos, however, where the scientific perspective and the goal of dominating nature rule, soul is considered a quaint idea that has outlived its usefulness.

Do we need the soul anymore for *any* purpose? Have healers throughout history had it wrong? Is there any reason for Grauds and Childers to be concerned about the soul's health in this book, or should the idea of the soul be consigned to the dustbin of history?

Invitations to the soul's funeral are premature. In fact, the evidence for the soul is stronger now than at any other time in human history because of a growing body of scientific data favoring the existence of an infinite, soul-like quality of human consciousness.[1] All told, this evidence suggests that human consciousness behaves *infinitely* in space and time—that it is not limited to specific points in space such as brains and bodies, and that it is not confinable to specific points in time such as the present.[2,3] In sum, these findings suggest that space and time are simply not applicable to certain operations of consciousness. Consciousness is *nonlocal;* it is both trans-spatial and trans-temporal; it is *not in* space and time. The implications are profound—for if something is nonlocal or infinite in space, it is omnipresent; and if nonlocal or infinite in time, it is eternal and immortal.[4] This nonlocal faculty of consciousness profoundly resembles what has been called the soul throughout human history.[5] Accompanying this evidence is a growing body of sophisticated hypotheses that may explain these phenomena.[6-10] Only by ignoring these developments can the soul be so breezily dismissed.

A growing number of scientists and researchers realize that consciousness and soul are not illusions, not merely brain-in-disguise.

Many now believe that consciousness is *fundamental* in the world and cannot be explained in terms of anything more basic.[11] Consciousness, in this view, is not manufactured by the brain and body, although it may work *through* them. As Nobel laureate in biology George Wald expresses the point, "Mind, rather than emerging as a late outgrowth in the evolution of life, has existed always..., the source and condition of physical reality."[12] Sir John C. Eccles, the Nobel laureate in neurobiology, adds, "I maintain that the human mystery is incredibly demeaned by scientific reductionism, with its claim to account for the entire spiritual world in terms of patterns of neuronal activity. This belief must be classed as a superstition. We have to recognize that we are spiritual beings with souls existing in a spiritual world as well as material beings with bodies and brains existing in a material world."[13] These scientists imply that Grauds and Childers are on solid ground in attending to the soul.

II.

To a shaman, as Grauds and Childers explain in the following pages, the diagnosis of many of our ailments is not difficult. The shaman would instantly recognize that we are suffering from *susto*—a loss of soul, a deadening of our individual and collective will, vision, and resolve, due in large measure to insecurity and fear.

It is fashionable to attribute this pervasive melancholy to the stresses of modern life and to the trauma inflicted by the terrorist attacks of September 11, but these are not the fundamental reasons that underlie our trepidations.

In spite of the threat of terrorism, we Americans have never lived more comfortably and securely than today, yet our fears are literally killing us. It isn't the big dreads such as another September 11 that are so debilitating, but the cumulative effect of the insidious little dreads that have become an accepted part of daily life. Consider the fact that more American males have their first heart attack on Monday morning, around 9 A.M., than at any other time of the week[14]—the so-called Black Monday syndrome—and that the level of job dissatisfaction in one's life is one of the best predictors of heart attack, right up there with blood pressure, smoking, cholesterol, and diabetes.[15] Consider too the Sisyphus Reaction, the "syndrome of joyless striving," named for the Greek mythological figure who was doomed forever to push a rock up a hill, only to have it slide down again.[16] Research shows that individuals who are engaged in joyless, psychologically stressful jobs in which they, like Sisyphus, cannot control their task and make no visible progress have an increased incidence of sudden cardiac death. As an antidote to the emptiness that is created by meaningless occupations, we are engaged in a national stampede to consume antidepressants and anti-anxiety drugs in record-busting quantities, without bothering to attend to the reasons why we need these substances in the first place.

Grauds and Childers provide an alternative to this approach—the realization of a spiritual dimension that can be called the "soul side" of life. It is from this dimension that an energized sense of meaning and purpose flows, without which life is empty and bland.

III.

Susto—soul loss—afflicts the most comfortable, secure, luxury-laden society that has ever existed. The hemorrhage of spirit, soul, and energy must be stanched if we are to recover our vitality as individuals and as a nation. Are we up to the task? I am an optimist on this question. The vigor that lies at the core of America's soul, which once stirred the hearts and hopes of the world, is not dead. But it is decidedly stunned by a new set of fears and by the dazzling promises of technology and the market, which suggest that the solution to our problems is to consume more and to medicate ourselves into an uncaring tranquillity to ease our nagging anxieties. Yet one of our most precious national traits endures—a deep-seated suspicion of artifice and false promises, and the capacity to identify matters of ultimate importance. Constance Grauds's and Douglas Childers's book is a wake-up call to what matters. It not only diagnoses a critical problem but offers elegant solutions as well. It is an invitation for every reader to perform a psycho-spiritual biopsy, assess her soul's health, and take whatever restorative measures may be needed. It is difficult to imagine what could be more important.

Larry Dossey, M.D.
Author of *Healing Beyond the Body, Reinventing Medicine*, and *Healing Words*

NOTES:

1. Dossey, Larry. The case for nonlocality. In: *Reinventing Medicine*. HarperSanFrancisco, 1999, pp. 37–84.
2. Olshansky, B.; Dossey, L. Retroactive prayer: A preposterous hypothesis? *British Medical Journal*. December 20, 2003; 327: 1465–68.
3. Braud, W. Wellness implications of retroactive intentional influence: exploring an outrageous hypothesis. *Alternative Therapies in Health & Medicine*. 2000; 6(1): 37–48.
4. Nadeau, Robert; Kafatos, Menas. *The Non-Local Universe: The New Physics and Matters of the Mind*. New York: Oxford University Press, 1999.
5. Dossey, Larry. *Recovering the Soul*. New York: Bantam Books, 1989.
6. Radin, Dean. Theory. In: *The Conscious Universe*. HarperSanFrancisco, 1997, pp. 277–87.
7. Dossey, Larry. Emerging theories. In: The return of prayer. *Alternative Therapies in Health and Medicine*. 1997; 3(6): 10–17, 113–20.
8. Brooks, M. The weirdest link: quantum entanglement. *New Scientist*. 27 March 2004, pp. 33–35.
   ———Vive la weirdness! Editorial on quantum entanglement, p. 3.
9. Atmanspacher, H.; Romer, H.; Walach, H. Weak quantum theory: complementarity and entanglement in physics and beyond. *Foundations of Physics*. 2002; 32: 379–406.
10. Clarke, C.J.S. The nonlocality of mind. *Journal of Consciousness Studies*. 1995; 2(3): 231–40.
11. Chalmers, D.J. The puzzle of conscious experience. *Scientific American*. 1995; 273(6): 80–86.

12. Wald, G. Quoted in: *Bulletin of the Foundation for Mind-Being Research*. September 1988: p. 3.

13. Eccles, J.C. *Evolution of the Brain, Creation of the Self*. New York: Routledge, 1991.

14. Dossey, Larry. Black Monday syndrome: When dread means dread. In: *Meaning & Medicine*. New York: Bantam Books, 1991, pp. 62–68.

15. *Work in America: Report of a Special Task Force to the Secretary of Health, Education, and Welfare*. Cambridge, MA: MIT Press, 1973.

16. Karasek, R.L.; Theorell, T.; Schwartz, J.E.; Schnall, P.L.; Pieper, C.F.; Michela, J.L. Job characteristics in relation to the prevalence of myocardial infarction. *American Journal of Public Health*. 1988; 78(8): 910–16.

The
Energy
Prescription

INTRODUCTION: Spirited Energy

by

Connie Grauds, R.Ph.

As a registered pharmacist, I dispense modern medicinal drugs to combat illness and alleviate afflictions of the body and the mind. As a shamana of Amazonian jungle tradition, I invoke the invisible medicine of the spirit to heal conditions of the mind, heart, and soul that often lie at the root of our bodily ailments. For shamans understand that spirit energy is the source of all life and vitality, in body, mind, and spirit.

Spirit energy, the vital force of life, is what we all desire and seek regardless of particular religious traditions or secular beliefs. Medical surveys show that "lack of energy" is the number-one complaint in physicians' offices today.

In the unusual course of my life's work I have sought to bridge two powerful medicine traditions. By integrating the spirit energy of shamanism with our modern health-care vision, a new level of sustainable health and vital energy, grounded in a vision of reciprocity and interdependence, is possible and available to all. The sustainable self described in this book naturally emerges from healing in relationship—with ourselves, with our family and our community, with nature, and with the Spirit of life itself that sustains us all.

My journey toward the health profession started in my early childhood, near one of Minnesota's famed 10,000 lakes. I was like any other good Catholic girl and ace student, except for one overwhelming secret: My mother heard voices, saw otherworldly visions, and spoke to apparitions. "Psychosis" was the term the doctors used for what other people called "crazy." And their prescribed "cure"—years of powerful drugs and electroshock treatments—reduced her to a haunted shadow of the person she had once been.

Being my mother's daughter, "going crazy" became my biggest fear. I compensated by excelling in math and science, whose cool objectivity, anchored in knowledge, facts, principles, and laws, promised control over the wildness of nature, life, and the very unpredictable human psyche. It seemed that a mind grounded in the sciences could never lose control. I graduated from the University of Minnesota's College of Pharmacy in 1969. I found a job as a health-care professional in an HMO. I married my college-town sweetheart. My life made sense. It seemed founded on unshakable ground.

For the next quarter of a century I was a practicing pharmacist. As a respected member of the medical community, I truly believed the high-tech pharmaceuticals I handed out would cure most ills. Over the years I filled hundreds of thousands of prescriptions. So many faces and names grew familiar as they came for endless refills year after year. Looking over the counter at these same customers asking for the same medications that had become their steady diet, I wondered, Are these drugs really helping? Are these people getting better? If I was really helping them, why did so many keep coming back? *Why were so many never cured?*

I was, and still am, aware of the fact that pharmaceutical drugs do help to alleviate suffering and facilitate healing for many. But I also began to notice that the pharmaceuticals I was dispensing often created dependency rather than true healing, and often generated side effects little better than the symptoms they were prescribed to alleviate. I became acutely aware of the fallacy of equating the suppression of symptoms with the curing of afflictions, or the absence of symptoms with genuine vitality and health. And my idealism and my faith in silver-bullet pharmaceuticals began to wane.

I also noticed something significant: Regardless of their ailments and medications, most of my customers over two and a half decades were complaining, in one way or another, of a lack of energy. They stood in line, lethargic, anxious, unhappy, depressed, often drinking coffee, grumbling over the side effects of the newest miracle drugs, waiting for refills of antibiotics, antidepressants, or tranquilizers. And their general complaints—fatigue, sleeplessness, depression, stress, anxiety, weight gain—boiled down to the same problem: loss of vitality. I grew tired of refilling prescriptions that alleviated symptoms while leaving people in states of diminished aliveness.

One day, in my early forties, I found myself on the other side of the counter, an anxious patient with a little lump on my throat. I was diagnosed with thyroid cancer. I had seen thousands of cancer patients over the years in every stage of the disease and the treatment, and I knew the physical and emotional devastation of both. Cancer is a brutal game of chance. As with Russian roulette, to win is to survive. Now I knew firsthand the fear and helplessness I had seen in countless cancer patients. They were in me. Facing the specter of death and disillusioned with Western medicine, I sank into the depths of a personal and a professional crisis.

Western medicine diagnosed and aggressively treated my condition and saved the life of my body. But it did not truly heal and revitalize me, or restore the aliveness I had lost somewhere along the way. It did not address the numerous underlying conditions and factors that preceded and perhaps contributed to my cancer. It did not address or alleviate the human fears that my cancer brought to a full boil—fears that remained after the diseased tissues were surgically removed and chemically bombarded from my body.

As I was gripped by those fears in my most vulnerable moments, Western medicine pointed me toward the path of medications that had made my mother a walking zombie. Medicating symptoms in the absence of addressing their root emotional and spiritual causes gives limbo, not life.

My cancer brought to my conscious awareness, now as a chronic experience, what shamans view as the root cause of all human afflictions: fear. I was living in fear. I was afraid of cancer as a malignant physical process; afraid of dying, afraid of surgery, afraid of physically devastating and uncertain chemotherapy, afraid of cancer returning even if my treatment was successful. And I saw that even before my cancer I had already been living in fear—of approaching middle age, of various physical ailments, of my disintegrating marriage, of my unsatisfying career. And I sensed deep, childhood fears that I had grown so used to I no longer noticed them and couldn't even identify them. To my dismay, after the cancer was removed from my body, the cancer of fear remained in me.

For months on end I experienced fear's effects and side effects: low energy, restlessness, anxiety, panic attacks, fatigue, depression, insomnia, a weakened immune system, and more. These emotional, physiological, and psychological conditions I had seen in countless patients over the years were now my own. And I no longer trusted the pharmacological solutions of my trade.

With my body and mind afflicted and my energy and aliveness draining away, my marriage of nearly twenty years ended and my life fell apart. I felt like dying, yet I wanted more than anything to *feel alive*. Then, through chance circumstances, I ended up in the depths of the Peruvian Amazon jungle, immersed in its multihued greens and its unbridled, primal aliveness. Within days I began to feel a deep calm and a renewed vitality. My true healing process had begun.

One night I found myself in a dim, smoke-filled hut, face-to-face with a jungle shaman. I had dealt with people at the top of their professions—high-powered doctors, surgeons, professors, educators, and hospital administrators. I had stared calmly across the pharmacy counter into the whirlpool eyes of psychotics, schizophrenics, and other troubled souls lost in the uncharted regions of the psyche. But I had never looked into eyes of such piercing depth as those of this simple jungle shaman.

Under the impact of his personal power—his jungle medicine—events took their own course. In that moment all the fear and helplessness rose up in me. I walked out of the hut after he finished his ritual and literally collapsed on the ground in an altered state of consciousness. That night I was plunged into the shaman's realm, a disorienting world of visions, energies, healing, and transformation. The encounter precipitated a journey that led me from the depths of my fear into the depths of my spirit.

I now see my painful crises, my disillusionment with Western medical methods and perspectives, and even my cancer, as blessings in disguise. They opened me to alternative healing visions and worldviews and led me to an extraordinary Amazon shaman, don Antonio. I would spend the next decade as his apprentice, immersing myself in the healing mysteries of native Amazon rain-forest shamanism. Under his guidance, shamanic disciplines, visions and experiences, and the jungle's natural, living pharmacopoeia became my course work and my textbooks. And on rare occasions, spirit entities literally became my personal physicians and teachers.

Gradually, over the course of my apprenticeship, I faced and healed the fears at the roots of my exhaustion, confusion, and illness and reclaimed my life. My shamanic training taught me things my Western medical training had not. I discovered that "my world" was largely a conditioned perceptual construct made of beliefs and interpretations used to limit the overwhelming flow of life within and around me. As new spiritual experiences and perceptions shifted or dissolved many of my seemingly solid beliefs, I learned to tap into and conduct nature's inexhaustible supply of spirit energy. In this process I recovered the radiant aliveness that is our birthright.

We are all interdependent beings designed to conduct spirit energy in all of our actions and relationships. The key to abundant energy is a natural, trusting, and balanced relationship with life in every area, including diet, breath, exercise, work, relaxation, sleep, play, human relationships, and more. Shamans call the basic areas of life the *entradas*, or gateways. And they say we access and conduct the spirit energy of life through these gateways.

Shamans tell us that a wellspring of limitless energy exists within us, even when we are ill or energy depleted. This book will teach you to access and conduct this energy within by managing the basic energy gateways in your life in very concrete and practical ways. And when that energy is unleashed in you, you will experience a new vitality and a freedom in your spirit, just as I did.

I now work as a shamanic healer in the Amazon and in America, while teaching the healing properties of natural medicines to Western health-care professionals. As a pharmacist and shamana I seek to integrate modern medicine's scientific knowledge and technological wizardry with "eco-medicine" or "spirited medicine." For Spirit is the ultimate medicine, the substance of all energy and the source of all healing. A complete healing paradigm must include Spirit, the soul, and the body and must address the deepest roots of illness and dis-ease.

Both traditional shamanism and modern psychology agree that the root of stress, lethargy, depletion, anxiety, depression, fatigue, despair, and a host of other familiar conditions is fear. Shamans call this energy-depleting, disease-producing fear *susto*, and they treat it like any other disease. And when we heal the roots of *susto* in us, we recover the vitality and aliveness that it stole from us.

The information, insights, and exercises in the following chapters will be useful to you whether or not you feel *susto* is a factor in your life. They will help you:

- Discern your energy leaks and their underlying causes.
- Discover how energy works in the various gateways of life.
- Understand these gateways as energy relationships, which can be as healthy or unhealthy as any other relationships.
- Examine, assess, and address each gateway's efficiency, or inefficiency, and see where and how you are dynamically conducting or leaking energy.
- Learn to access spirit energy directly, relieve anxiety and stress, recharge your body and mind with vitality, and "up your energy voltage."
- Design an energy prescription for life that addresses your own needs and issues in all of the gateways.

My co-author, Doug Childers, and I hope you will use this book to reclaim the vitality and radiant aliveness that you were born with. Limitless energy is available for everyone to have a healthy, productive life full of vitality, meaning, passion, love, and joy. It is possible to create such a life for yourself. It is already yours in potential, and by design.

Now let's take a closer look at energy from a shamanic perspective to see what it is, where it comes from, how it "works," and more.

Section One

Personal Energy Crisis:
Old Paradigm Problem,
New Paradigm Solution

1

The Quest for More Energy: Are You Winning or Losing the Energy Game?

The search for energy is the American Dream that never sleeps. Everyone wants more of it, and most people feel like they can't get enough of it. In our pursuit of energy we may take up—for a while—demanding diets, exercise programs, and expensive vitamin and supplement regimes.

But the path to abundant energy is not product related. It is not achieved through extreme efforts or eccentric programs that prey on your fears or promote obsessive concerns about fitness, diet, and health. It is a path of balance, sanity, and intelligent self-effort that supports the most complex and demanding life and leads you into simple and direct relationship with your self and the Source of life. Health and vitality require proper energy management and are a by-product of it.

In nature, the basic life processes occur without confusion or dilemma. For most life-forms, managing energy is as simple as breathing fresh air, absorbing sunlight, foraging for food, resting, reproducing, living, and dying within an interdependent web of life.

Ancient shamans observed these natural processes and extracted simple principles that allowed them to acquire and conduct far greater amounts of energy than the average person. By under-standing and managing the simple life processes and natural forces to which all creatures are subject and using their own bodies and minds as laboratories, they achieved personal energy mastery. And they shared their knowledge, or "medicine," with their village or tribe.

But in our modern world, with its stressful pace and complexity, the basic life processes have become complicated, confusing, and riddled with dilemma. The body operates 24/7, waking and sleep-ing, without our effort. Disconnected from nature and alienated from our natural or "indigenous" self that intuitively knows what it needs, simple functions like diet, exercise, sex, and breathing may seem like near-impenetrable mysteries. So we turn to experts to un-derstand, and hopefully meet, our most basic human needs.

We've acquired remarkable scientific knowledge about diet, ex-ercise, sex, the brain, meditation and prayer, and more. But what are the fundamentals of human energy that, if applied, allow us to be-come revitalized energy beings? Here traditional shamanic wisdom is still relevant to modern life. The shamanic energy principles pre-sented in this book confirm insights in modern psychology, modern physics, and modern scientific research. And no matter how com-plex the world becomes, our bodies, our minds, our relationships, and our vital energy systems will always operate on the same time-less principles.

The modern rush-hour lifestyle leaves millions too depleted to get sufficient exercise, relaxation, play, or even spend quality time with their families. This energy-depleting lifestyle can lead to chronic stress, anxiety, fatigue, high blood pressure, depression, insomnia, a weakened immune system, and a host of serious physical and psy-chological ailments.

Energy depletion is an inevitable result of unresolved life stress combined with common neglect. In our often anxious efforts to keep up the pace, we fail to do many simple, basic things that maintain our vital connection to the source of abundant energy that sustains us. And this matter of stress and anxiety is key.

The Wages of Fear

Today, frequent "orange alerts" and scare reports send anxiety rippling through our culture, increasing our stress, depleting our energy, and undermining our health and well-being. But even before the shocking events of 9/11 inaugurated an "era of terror," nearly two-thirds of Americans were chronically under stress and sleep deprived, 40 percent experienced significant daytime tiredness, 60 percent suffered recurring fatigue, 65 million experienced anxiety, and 17.5 million adults experienced depression.

We are encouraged to seek energy and health in a cup, a serum, or a pill. Two of America's top-grossing drugs in 2003 were the popular antidepressants Zoloft and Prozac.

Natural energy- and health-supplement sales are up by 15 percent. Consumption of artificial energy boosters is at an all-time high. And coffee shops spring up across America like mushrooms after rain. But quick-fix energy substitutes and symptom-suppressing drugs cannot solve our long-term energy and health needs.

The cause of most enervation, depletion, and fatigue illness is not a lack of energy, but a life lived out of balance. This is true for an individual, a family, a nation, or a planet. To a shaman, depletion and fatigue are signs that we are habitually disconnecting from the limitless supply of energy that sustains us, or we are habitually obstructing or "leaking" the energy we have.

Call it chi, manna, spirit, prana, vitality, or Light; view it through the lens of shamanism, ancient spiritual teachings, modern medicine, or quantum physics—energy is the stuff of life, the ultimate medicine, the Holy Grail we're all seeking. No one knows exactly what it is, but everyone knows it when they feel it. We know instinctively that our health, vitality, happiness, productivity, clarity, creativity, sexuality, longevity, and more depend on how much energy we have. And we know that the more energy we have, the better we feel.

Energy level is an indicator of our general health. A Yale University study found that energy levels had the highest correlation with general-health status and were the best predictor of both physical and psychological health over time. Energetic people, the study showed, are generally healthy, whereas the enervated are often ill, becoming ill, fighting off illness, or struggling with their low-energy condition. Illness, apathy, fatigue, anxiety, chronic stress, depression, and the like are all signs that we are losing the energy game.

The Western Fallacy of Pharmaceutical Healing

Nearly three decades in the trenches of Western medicine and a personal health crisis taught me firsthand that medications and operations do not cure fear, generate energy, or produce vibrant health. Those suffering chronic low energy and poor health who look to conventional Western medicine to restore their full vitality and aliveness are doomed to disappointment for the following reasons:

Conventional medicine is typically passive and remedial rather than dynamically proactive. Doctors give you things to take, and do things to you. But vitality is a result of a dynamic, proactive lifestyle.

Conventional medicine views the body mechanistically and treats it in mechanical and chemical terms, rather than in energetic and holistic terms. The body is an admittedly marvelous biochemical machine. But energy is *not* generated through mechanical or chemical medical procedures.

Conventional medicine generally ignores or denies the spiritual dimensions of sickness and health. And many recent scientific studies demonstrate that patients with deep spiritual beliefs tend to be healthier, happier, and better at dealing with stress.

Conventional medicine has tended to be remedial rather than proactive. Doctors give you things to take and treat your body to make you well after you are sick. Now forward-thinking clinicians are beginning to recommend lifestyle changes, knowing that health and vitality are a result of a dynamic, proactive lifestyle.

Not long ago we entered the era of holistic medicine, the consideration of the whole person—a big step. Now it's time for holistic medicine to join up with energy medicine, spirited medicine, which is the medicine of the future.

Psychopharmacological prescription medications have helped millions of people with serious emotional or psychological disorders, but they can hardly be said to have *healed* them. These medications can seem to be a godsend, offering quick relief by suppressing, diminishing, and even eliminating painful or debilitating symptoms. But in our pharmaceutical culture, too many doctors prescribe these medications, and too many patients reach for them, in knee-jerk fashion.

Pharmaceuticals temporarily diminish anxiety, panic, and depression; decrease our emotional and physical pain; or kill hostile germs in the body. Yet they leave the root causes of our ailments untouched and diminish our capacity to feel. And our feelings contain vital information that is essential for our health, well-being, and peak functioning.

The containment, suppression, or elimination of unpleasant symptoms does not produce vitality or health. The real healing solutions lie in the realms of spirit and nature. To heal an unbalanced, stressful, or fragmented life, we must consistently access the life-sustaining sources of spirit energy.

Most preventable illness is a by-product of energy-depleting habits and behaviors that are driven by unhealthy thinking and emotional patterns. So healing also necessarily involves a change in consciousness.

By focusing primarily on symptoms and pathologies, Western medicine, even at its breathtaking best, remains an exalted science of damage control that cannot produce the radiant aliveness that most of us experienced in childhood. And that is what we instinctively long for.

We Are Nature's Most Advanced Energy Conductors

Human beings are sophisticated organic energy systems participating in a complex relationship with the ultimate energy system of Life, which includes all of nature and the entire cosmos. All living things expend and receive energy with every breath, bite, movement, impulse, perception, and sensation. Everything that exists and all actions and events in the universe are energetic phenomena. Psychologist Carl Jung's assertion that every experience and event in our life and in our psyche has an energetic value and impact confirms a principle shamans have long known.

Shamans view all states as energy states and see all interactions between us and the world as forms of spirit energy exchange. They know that our healing and vital aliveness depend on our relationship with the natural, vibrant, regenerative processes through which we conduct spirit energy. This worldview is compatible with current quantum physics' views of the universe as a vast, interconnected, living sea of subatomic particles and waves of light and energy at times appearing as matter.

Yet if we are literally made of, and are living within, a limitless sea of light and energy, how can we suffer chronic low energy, fatigue, or poor health? Shamans say the root of illness and enervation is a subtle, primal fear, which they call *susto*. And they treat it like any health condition. In the next chapter we'll look at fear from both shamanic and contemporary Western psychological perspectives, which are surprisingly parallel.

2

Susto: The Root of Energy Depletion

Is there a root cause of low energy, poor health, and emotional, physical, or spiritual disease? Western medicine says no. Amazon shamans say there is, and point to a condition or negative "spirit" called *susto.* To shamans, *susto* is "the worm at the core" of all suffering and disease. It is the "sickness of fear" that separates us from the Source of spirit energy and from our own soul or essential self.

Susto is a spiritual affliction that leads to a host of physical, psychological, and spiritual ailments. It devours our life force, distorts our perceptions, affects our functioning and our relationships, weakens our immune system, and renders us vulnerable to afflictions of every kind. Amazon shamans view low energy, apathy, anxiety, depression, and most physical ailments as secondary effects of *susto,* so they treat it at the first signs of its appearance.

Shamans speak of the "spirit of" a condition or an illness. Western medicine speaks of causes and symptoms. Both are metaphors of choice for two different healing paradigms. Yet if you've ever been truly frightened or "in the grip of fear," you'll appreciate the shaman's view of *susto* as "possession by the spirit of fear."

Shamans know that the hidden spiritual roots of any ailment must be addressed, not just the visible branches or outer symptoms that catch our attention. Seeing illness as a spiritual affliction and seeing healing as a restoration of the patient's soul or true self, they treat a person's spirit as well as his or her body. They know that the release from *susto* that reconnects us to our soul, our essential self, and the source of our life requires a shift in consciousness.

Western medicine can measure the biochemical effects of fear on the nervous system and the body and mind, but it cannot tell us what fear ultimately *is,* let alone what the soul is. Yet, however you define it, traditional shamans and Western medicine and psychology know that chronic fear can cost us our peace of mind, our health, our sanity, and our aliveness.

When don Antonio first told me about *susto,* it sounded like primitive superstition to my Western ears.

"But don Antonio," I argued, "fear is one of the most common human feelings. Everyone experiences fear from time to time. What is there to treat, unless it becomes anxiety, or panic, or depression, or triggers a physical illness?"

He seemed genuinely puzzled by my argument. Finally, he said, "Connie, is it wisdom to wait for *susto* to produce secondary effects, and then just treat the effects?"

Put like that, it was a no-brainer. Don Antonio then explained the nature of *susto.* It can be triggered by an accident, an emotional shock, perceived danger, verbal or physical abuse, threat of abandonment or rejection, and other events. Chronic stress is already *susto,* eating away at the core of our life energy. He used the example of a jaguar in the jungle. If a jaguar crosses your path, fear gives you energy to take appropriate action, like running away. But once you've taken action and you're out of danger, it doesn't help to keep re-imagining the event, or to imagine the jaguar actually eating you. To keep fear alive in your mind and your body is *susto*.

Don Antonio said *susto* is easily remedied when treated early on. But if left untreated, it can develop into more serious conditions over time. It can become a habit that changes and may even define our personality. It can also be transmitted to others like any contagious disease.

Don Antonio told me, "Think of a time you were with someone who was anxious, upset, or fearful, or even happy or peaceful. Do you recall how you felt their feelings in a sympathetic response?"

I recalled attending a college football game and how easily I became swept up in the emotions of the crowd. Don Antonio said that we absorb each other's energetic and emotional conditions, positive and negative, because we are energetically connected. The spread of *susto* is as real as the spread of a flu virus—and it is just as depleting.

Even Western medicine knows that chronic fear depletes our energy, that even low-grade fear or anxiety lowers our immune system over time, and that this makes us vulnerable to physical and emotional ailments. So recognizing *susto* as an energy-depleting spiritual condition that can cause physical, emotional, and psychological harm is common sense. It allows us to examine and address our fears in healthy ways long before they cost us our health or well-being.

I now know that in my years as a pharmacist I saw thousands of undiagnosed cases of *susto*, many of which had progressed to far worse conditions. But like the doctors who wrote the prescriptions I filled, I was completely focused on the secondary symptoms, the physical and psychological ailments. I know that I also suffered from *susto* for years. And by ignoring it, I was unable to address effectively the physical, emotional, and psychological afflictions to which it contributed, including my cancer.

Mood-suppressing, mind-altering drugs like Xanax, Prozac,

Paxil, Zoloft, Ritalin, and Valium are commonly prescribed for disorders like anxiety, panic, insomnia, depression, hyperactivity, and ADS. Yet the low-grade chronic fear that underlies and often precedes such conditions is ignored, and is often called boredom or restlessness. And the varied life circumstances underlying these conditions are also often left out of the equation in the pharmaceutical approach.

Many doctors automatically write pharmaceutical prescriptions for physical, emotional, and spiritual ailments. But to treat with drugs *susto's* secondary symptoms and effects is to prune the branches of our afflictions while ignoring the roots from which they spring. And the short-term "solutions" pharmaceuticals offer frequently come with long-term costs.

For shamans, *susto* marks the beginning of the loss of self that leaves us vulnerable to accidents, physical and psychological illness, and ultimately death. So they treat it at its first appearance, and it seems to work. Most indigenous peoples I've spent time with whose cultures are still intact are notable for a lack of restlessness, stress, anxiety, depression, obesity, and a host of other modern afflictions. And they are notable for their general cheerfulness, well-being, and vitality, and their remarkable intimacy with nature.

Modern Westerners, on the other hand, are largely *susto*-driven, often harried, anxious, worried, restless, impatient, and in a hurry. Separated from the earth by layers of asphalt and cement, we are like infants in sterile incubators craving nourishing contact with the mother, craving her warmth, her smell, and the primal beating of her heart.

Shamans view the prevalence of *susto*-based maladies like stress, anxiety, depression, ADS, and chronic fatigue in Western culture as a result of this physical and emotional disconnection from nature, and from our own indigenous self-nature.

Two Selves, Two Options

Modern psychology confirms traditional shamanic wisdom when it posits fear as a fundamental force in the human psyche and a primal human drive. The primal fear of modern psychology, the existential dread of Kierkegaard, and the *susto* of Amazon shamanism are the same. Søren Kierkegaard, Sigmund Freud, Otto Rank, Carl Jung, Ernest Becker, Alice Miller, and numerous other pioneers of the psyche—modern Western shamans—all point to this fear as the grain of sand around which the mysterious pearl of human personality forms as a necessary social and survival tool and as a psychological shelter and defense against the storms of living.

It will be useful to summarize some fundamental insights of modern psychology that corroborate shamanic perspectives on energy depletion and energy rejuvenation and lay the groundwork for some of the key metaphors we will be using in this book, particularly what we call here the "*susto* self" and the "indigenous self." (For a profound and comprehensive overview of these and other matters, we highly recommend the works of Ernest Becker and Alice Miller, in particular Becker's *Denial of Death* and Miller's *Thou Shalt Not Be Aware*.)

Indigenous cultures are not devoid of unhealthy stresses and flaws, but they have remarkable natural and spiritual characteristics that modern cultures lack. Let's briefly explore these two selves and their origins in the light of modern psychology, and see how each one shapes our character and mediates our connection to the life force that sustains us.

The complex modern personality is both an evolutionary development in the life of consciousness in the universe and an unhealthy distortion of the indigenous self that each of us is at birth. We are, at birth, nature's cutting-edge design, possessing the most sophisticated intelligence on the planet, and we are also as primal as a tiger cub, a fawn, or an eagle hatchling. But through the complex socializing process, we become "products" of modern culture, which overvalues the personality and undervalues the indigenous self and its mysterious inner life.

These two selves—the indigenous self we are at birth and the complex socialized personality we become over time—represent two life streams and two ways of being in the world. Each self has its strengths and weaknesses, and both are necessary. We cannot wholly sacrifice one to the other. And we must integrate these two selves in order to fulfill our human potential and our evolutionary purpose, in order to become truly *sustainable selves* capable of creating a sustainable world.

All infants experience relatively unimpeded access to the vital energy that sustains them. They live in primal contact with nature through their feelings, impulses, perceptions, and relationships. The infant's marvelous vital intensity and the joyous, uninhibited play of young children demonstrate the incredible life energy that is meant to flow through us all. Children live in this flow as long as their vital needs are met, their natural life expressions are accepted, and they are loved, respected, cared for, and are protected from danger, pain, and trauma.

From infancy on, each of us undergoes a process of systematic indoctrination that turns us into socialized personalities. This process includes a combination of rewards and punishments, positive and negative feedback. Sadly, the human "system" we all depend upon inevitably fails and betrays us in countless ways. Our childhood experiences may include love, tenderness, kindness, praise, and support. But they may also include punishment, criticism, rejection, abandonment, coercion, emotional, physical or sexual abuse, the breaking of our will, illness, accidents, and other difficulties. And the worst of these occurrences may be carried out with the best of intentions.

Our personality is formed before puberty by all of the above, as well as by prenatal, genetic, and other mysterious factors. Add to this the natural fear that every helplessly dependent infant experiences in a world of greater, mysterious, and at times frightening powers. The increasing and necessary defenses and adaptations to life in an unpredictable and at times threatening world solidify our human personality and progressively distance us from our indigenous self. Thus each of us gradually becomes, to one degree or another, a *susto* self in a *susto* world.

Modern psychology has much to say about the formation of human personality and the socialization and indoctrination process in which it occurs. The various aims of child-rearing are to protect and nurture us, to mold us and develop our character, to teach us essential life skills, to make us obedient and easier to manage for our parents' convenience and the needs of our culture, and for numerous other purposes that vary from family to family and culture to culture.

This process produces mixed results. We become proficient and complex personalities in a socialized world, but our indigenous self is mostly lost to us and our access to its extraordinary intuitive and physical gifts, its dynamic vitality, and its innate connection to nature are severely diminished.

The indigenous self, with its boundless energy, intuitive perceptions, and feeling sensitivity to life, is essential for our well-being, vitality, and wholeness. To the degree that we lose touch with this self, we experience confusion in our relationships with others and with life; our basic needs, feelings, and appetites become complicated; and our relationship to the energy gateways becomes stressful and problematic. The loss of this indigenous self is the source of most of the ailments, neuroses, and pathologies that plague modern Western man.

So what is the solution? Albert Einstein's insight that "no problem is solved by the same consciousness that created it" affirms what deep shamanism, modern psychology, and many spiritual traditions know: Finding solutions to our problems requires a change in our consciousness. This book views this shift in consciousness as a recovery of the indigenous self that restores our vital connection to life.

The Fear That Ails Us,
the Medicine That Heals Us

In the spring of 2002 I was in a small remote village on the Yarapa River, a day's journey south of the jungle town of Iquitos in the northern Peruvian Amazon rain forest. I had come to this village as a shamana, by invitation of shaman don Antonio with whom I had apprenticed for the past ten years. During my two-week stay don Antonio and I would treat local villagers for a variety of conditions and ailments—physical, mental, emotional, and spiritual—while we continued our shamanic work together.

I had brought a kit with traditional pharmaceutical supplies, such as bandages, antibiotics, aspirin, hydrogen peroxide, and other useful essentials. But my primary medicines would be natural and my primary methods shamanic, both having their origins in the jungle's overwhelming surplus and pharmacopoeia of spirit energy.

On the second morning of my visit, a young village woman in her mid-teens named Maria came to my hut for a healing. In my previous visit there six months earlier she had been my cook. Maria now had a one-month-old daughter who needed a healing. When I asked her what was wrong with her little girl, she said her daughter had *susto* and often awakened crying in fear during the night.

I asked Maria the usual questions any Western medical practitioner would ask—about the overall physical health of her child and herself, about any unusual conditions, changes, or events that might be causing her daughter's *susto*. Her answers gave me no clear indication of any specific causes. I told Maria to come back that afternoon with her daughter.

The heat of the midday tropical sun bore down as Maria entered my hut a few hours later, now holding her new baby. Her young husband and her mother were with her. After greeting them, I examined the infant while making "you adorable baby" talk, rubbing her cheeks, smoothing her forehead, squeezing her little hands, and looking into her beautiful brown eyes. She was restless and lethargic, not a happy, healthy baby.

Then I spoke with the three adults for a few moments, observing them closely. Both parents seemed apprehensive and concerned. The grandmother, clearly upset, pointed repeatedly at her little granddaughter with an unpleasant, agitated expression, saying, "This child is not normal!" She was a one-woman *susto* generator. Her method of dealing with her fear seemed to be blaming others, which is also a method of transmitting *susto*!

Doctors who focus on their patient's extended family do their patients a huge service. For every patient is a part of a larger whole, interdependent with and unavoidably affected by a complex web of human circumstances and relationships. One cannot effectively treat a patient as a separate unit. These complex influences must be taken into account. And in this baby's case, the family dynamic was an important factor.

Next I performed a healing ceremony I had learned from don Antonio. I lit a *mapacho* tobacco cigarette and began to sing *icaros*—sacred healing songs—over the child while blowing the ritual tobacco smoke gently over her listless head. This soothing ritual, which

invokes the tangible healing presence and energy of Spirit, has par-
allels in many ancient spiritual and healing traditions. Within moments her little face grew peaceful, and her droopy eyes soon closed
in restful sleep. But the session was not over. The others were still
visibly anxious. Was their *susto* about the baby? Had the baby picked
up their *susto*? I couldn't tell. But clearly the whole family was in
susto.

I next performed a healing on Maria. She was completely receptive and grateful. She knew she had *susto,* and she trusted me. After
her, I approached her young husband. He sat slumped uncomfort-
ably in a chair, round-shouldered and staring at the floor, looking
defeated, ashamed, and worried about his baby. I sensed that he
was ashamed at the idea that he might have fathered a defective
child. I could see that his *susto,* combined with his helplessness and
shame, was concocting a case of depression.

I began the ritual. Within minutes he straightened up and began
taking deep, invigorating breaths. Soon the dullness in his eyes was
gone, replaced by a sparkle of alertness. I felt surges of spirit energy
flowing through his body, opening the blocks in him caused by his
fear.

Finally I went to the grandmother, who I sensed was the main
susto carrier in the family. A simple healing for a baby girl had turned
into a family affair! After I worked with the grandmother for five or
ten minutes, she finally calmed down. Then, as they all sat quietly in
the shade of my little hut with the baby suckling peacefully at her
mother's breast, I gave them my diagnosis and prescription.

"There is nothing wrong with this child except for the *susto,*" I
told them gently but with my shaman's authority. "So you must accept her fully into your heart and your home. All of you come back
for healing every day for the next week. Your child will grow
stronger. There is nothing to fear. You have been blessed with a

beautiful baby. She has the soul of an angel. Just love her with all your heart and everything will be fine."

They all seemed very relieved. They smiled, watching the baby nursing peacefully at Maria's breast. Through ritual, invocation, and relationship, I had enabled them to make a shift in consciousness, from the *susto* self to the indigenous self, and their connection to spirit energy, the power that heals, was restored. They had come fixated and isolated in fear, disconnected from relationship with themselves and each other. My ritual helped to magnify spirited energy, to reassure them that all was well, to return their attention to the bonds of love that tied them together as a family. As a result the "spell" of *susto* was broken and a very real and meaningful healing was accomplished.

In an American clinic this scene might have played out very differently. The little girl's fear might not have been recognized and treated. The anxious family would not have been brought into the healing circle. They might all have left in more or less the same state in which they arrived. The baby would have gone home to the same environment that had bred the *susto*, perhaps with a pharmaceutical prescription. And the *susto*, untreated and perhaps even aggravated by any prescribed medications, might develop into other physical, emotional, psychological, or spiritual conditions.

As a shaman, I view the people who come to me for help as energetic, spiritual beings who happen to live in bodies. I look for and treat *susto* in them, which is usually there. To soothe and calm them is sometimes enough to restore their connection to their own spirit so they can tap into the spirit energy that is within and all around them. A healing relationship between a doctor and a patient involves a direct exchange of spirit energy through attention, presence, trust, and compassion or love. And any relationship that embodies these qualities is a healing relationship that is grounded in the spirit, and in the indigenous self.

THE FOUR CATEGORIES OF FEAR

The following four basic types of fear, from subliminal to extreme, are a part of our human condition and operate to some degree in all of us, robbing us of energy and freedom:

Social or shame-based fear. This includes fear of rejection, of judgment, of failure, of seeming foolish, of being unworthy, of not fitting in, of being wrong. Its primal origins are the fears of social ostracism, tribal banishment, and of being shunned or exiled from one's community.

Fear of no control. This includes fear of one's surroundings or circumstances, fear of the actions and motives and behavior of others, and, ultimately, fear of a world that is felt, experienced, or perceived to be unpredictable, unreliable, or dangerous. To the degree that this fear lives in us, we contract emotionally, tense up physically, think obsessively, mistrust life, and are consciously or unconsciously driven by concerns for self-protection, personal safety, and the meeting of basic needs.

Fear of death and dying. This fear is first noticed as a fear for one's own physical safety, health, well-being, or, by extension, the safety and well-being of loved ones. One may consciously fear death when there is no apparent reason for such a fear. In its extreme, one may feel literal gut-wrenching, blood-chilling, paralyzing terror in the face of imminent or potential death or horrific physical injury. Those who have experienced this know that these phrases are not metaphors, but visceral effects.

Existential dread. This fourth fear is the most basic and least acknowledged in Western medicine. It is the root *susto* of the shamans that underlies all human anxiety. It is the fear modern psychology points to at the core of most human anxiety and neurosis. It is a primal fear of being separated from the Source of life, God, the ocean of spirit energy that sustains all living things. More than a fear of death, existential dread is a fear of ultimate extinction, meaningless existence, cosmic alienation, or eternal damnation. Most religious, magical, primitive, or superstitious rituals and practices are humans' attempts to banish, solve, or assuage this primal fear by appeasing, pleasing, invoking the blessing, or winning the favor of real or imagined supernatural forces or powers.

Having examined the *susto* self and its defining fears, we will now examine a sustainable energy paradigm that holds the keys to an energy-efficient, energy-abundant life.

3

A Sustainable Self

The key to abundant energy is not more information funneled into an already overloaded brain, a lengthy to-do list added to an already hectic life, or a sum of positive behaviors and habits. The key is a shift in consciousness that opens you up to new understandings and greater energy that you then conduct in the gateways.

And this shift in consciousness deepens *your understanding* of energy and *your relationship* to the Source of it.

According to modern physicists and ancient sages, every atom in the universe, and within us, is charged with dynamic energy. Split an atom and enough energy is released to destroy a major city! Everything, including us, is made of energy. Our every molecule, cell, feeling, perception, action, and experience is an expression of pure energy. In reality, we live in a sea of limitless energy. But until we learn to manage the stresses of life effectively—which is the essence of energy management—we may periodically, or chronically, become enervated and depleted.

Abundant vitality flows from our healthy functioning in the energy gateways of diet, work, breath, hydration, exercise, sexuality, relationships, and reciprocity. The gateways are the spokes of your energy wheel. Spirit is the hub. But in *susto,* the gateways are often sources of stress and energy leaks rather than sources of vitality and rejuvenation. And the difference begins in the mind.

Both illness and health begin with thoughts and feelings that either rejuvenate or deplete your energy and strengthen or weaken your immune system. Energy-depleting thoughts and feelings underlie energy-depleting habits. That external factors may contribute to an illness doesn't change the fact that sickness and health *always begin and end inside of you.*

Effective energy management begins in the mind, where we learn to shift from the *susto* self to the indigenous self. In *susto,* we struggle with the forces of life, trapped in the consciousness that creates our problems and energy-depleting habits and behaviors. At best we wrestle with habits and behaviors, trying to stop or change "bad" ones and create and sustain "good" ones. But we are unable to manage effectively what is going on inside of us because we are anxiously focused on what is happening outside of us. So in *susto* our energy and stress levels are primarily determined by what is going on around us and in our lives.

A Sustainable Self

When we reconnect to our indigenous self and make it the basis of effective energy-management skills, we begin to develop a *sustainable self.* What are the characteristics of a sustainable self? A sustainable self recognizes and embraces its interdependent relationship to life. This interdependence is evidenced by the fact that we live from breath to breath, that our life depends upon nature and the earth for food and resources and upon our cooperation with numerous interdependent beings like ourselves.

By embracing our interdependence in the web of life, we become receptive to the limitless energy that sustains all of creation. By living in dynamic cooperation with life via the gateways—by consistently doing things that replenish and heal us and not doing things that needlessly exhaust and deplete us—we access and conduct the energy we need to make and sustain positive changes and function at peak levels. And this naturally fills us with vitality and joy.

The "trick," then, is how to get from our *susto* self to a sustainable self and function there consistently.

How to Get from Here to There

"No problem is solved by the same consciousness that created it."
—**Albert Einstein**

Einstein, a modern quantum sage, recognized that a solution to a problem requires a shift in consciousness. Shamans know that the shift from the problematic *susto* self to the solution-oriented sustainable self also requires a change of consciousness. Shamans always seek solutions through a shift in consciousness. They achieve this shift through simple disciplines that increase their capacity to conduct spirit energy. These disciplines are the foundation of effective energy management.

A partial list of effective disciplines includes exercise, breathing, conscious relaxation, meditation, prayer, sacred ritual, meaningful work, selfless service, deep emotional contact with others, and being in nature. There are also "not doing" disciplines, like celibacy, fasting and dietary restrictions, and periods of withdrawal from the stimulation of the world into silence or solitude.

Such disciplines purify and focus the mind, shift your consciousness, release stress, raise your energy level, trigger new insights and perspectives, and increase your capacity to receive and conduct spirit energy. These disciplines do not depend upon particular religious or metaphysical beliefs to be effective.

The shift into the indigenous self is the most important discipline there is. It is the shift in consciousness we have been discussing. In this shift you consciously relax, release stress, and enter a state of calm yet heightened awareness that is profoundly restful, energizing, and rejuvenating.

With practice, this simple discipline becomes a natural response to stress that allows you to manage and transform your inner life before your outer circumstances change. It isn't always possible to remove or "fix" an outer problem immediately. You can't always quit your job, resolve a troubled relationship, change your children's behavior, heal a serious injury or disease, or eliminate stressful problems like noisy neighbors, rush-hour traffic, a bad economy, social injustice, world hunger, terrorism, poverty, and war.

But you *can* change your state of consciousness and deal effectively with the stresses and problems in your life, whatever they may be. And when you know how to do this, your fate will be—as it always has been—in your own very capable hands.

Section Two

The Eight Gateways to Energy

4

The Mind/Soul Gateway:
The Shift to the Sustainable Self

Wherever a thought goes, a chemical goes with it.... Your cells are constantly processing experience and metabolizing it according to your personal views.... Someone who is depressed over losing his job projects sadness everywhere in his body—the brain's output of neurotransmitters becomes depleted, hormone levels drop, the sleep cycle is interrupted, neuro-peptide receptors on the outer surface of skin cells become distorted, platelet cells in the blood become stickier and more prone to clump, and even his tears contain different chemical traces than tears of joy.... This point reinforces the great need to use our awareness to create the bodies we actually want.

—**Deepak Chopra**, *Ageless Body, Timeless Mind*

The mind is our soul's consciousness, our window of awareness to both the inner and outer worlds. It is the customs agent for all of the information, stimuli, and experience that continually bombard us from birth to death. It uses the brain to perceive, process, and comprehend visual and sensory stimuli, information, ideas, and impressions. The brain links the mind and the body, and enables the mind to exercise its will in the physical world.

Perceiving or thinking and breathing are the only involuntary functions subject to voluntary control. We control the mind by directing our attention and to some extent choosing the thoughts we think and the images, information, and stimuli we let in. Disciplines like meditation, prayer, and conscious relaxation are forms of mind management. Their purpose is to shift our consciousness from *susto* into higher states of awareness. But the primary shift in awareness takes us into the indigenous self.

The stressful thoughts that lead to the secretion of stress-related norepinephrine impede our evolutionary-derived natural healing capacities. These thoughts are often only in our minds, not a reality.

—**Dr. Herbert Benson**, president of Harvard
Medical School's Mind/Body Medical Institute

Recent technological innovations have allowed us to examine the molecular basis of the emotions, and to begin to understand how the molecules of our emotions share intimate connections with, and are indeed inseparable from, our physiology. . . . Consciously or, more frequently, unconsciously, we choose how we feel at every single moment.

—**Dr. Candice Pert**, neuroscientist, *The Molecules of Emotion*

Current neuroscience has proven that our thoughts, beliefs, and emotions affect our bodies at a cellular and chemical level, significantly affecting energy and health. An undisciplined mind leaks vital energy in a continuous stream of thoughts, worries, and skewed perceptions, many of which trigger disturbing emotions and degenerative chemical processes in the body.

The *susto* self thrives in a mind habitually involved in anxious, compulsive, and unproductive thinking. The sustainable self observes and manages the mind. It consciously relaxes and releases

negative habitual thinking. It directs its attention to respor
priately to situations rather than to react unconsciously in
a key element in this process of mind management is someunng
called *somatic awareness*.

Somatic awareness is the highly sophisticated, nonrational, sensory and emotional intelligence of the body and mind. Most of us
have enough somatic awareness to feel cold and heat, hunger and
fullness, pleasure and pain, sadness and happiness. Studies show
that when we eat with somatic awareness and savor the taste of our
food, our bodies absorb more of its nutrients. When we engage life
in the same way, we derive more energy, insight, meaning, and joy
from our experience.

Deep somatic awareness calms and heals the mind and emotions. It draws spirit energy into the body, charging the cells and tissues with life force. It releases stress and accelerates recovery from
the negative physical and emotional impact of experience. With a
few minutes of daily practice, our somatic awareness can be honed
into a highly refined awareness that is emotional and physical, practical and spiritual. Shamans develop this to a degree that allows
them to function at peak levels and to access extraordinary states of
consciousness.

All of us were born with a highly refined somatic awareness. It
was our primary medium of perception in the womb and in our
early infancy. But we unconsciously and progressively suppressed
this sensitivity in order to avoid feeling fear, pain, and other uncomfortable emotions and sensations.

This suppression of feeling-awareness, a kind of involuntary
and habitual psychic flinch, is the *susto* self's defining activity. It
seems to give temporary relief from stress and to protect us from the
increasing stimuli bombardment and information overload of our
modern technological world. But it diminishes our ability to perceive,

interpret, and integrate life's complex multisensory stimuli. It diminishes our emotional intelligence and our capacity for intimacy and relationship. It diminishes our ability to relax and release stress, ensuring our downward slide into states of energy depletion. And it diminishes our capacity to receive and digest the spirit energy on which our vitality and health depend.

Chronic somatic suppression is a serious handicap in life that leads to negative domino effects. Accumulated stress and tension floods our body with toxic chemicals, constricts our breathing, limits our oxygen and our energy intake, weakens our immune system, and makes us vulnerable to countless ailments, afflictions, and diseases.

> *The human brain has about 100,000,000,000 (100 billion)*
> *neurons, and about 1,000,000,000,000,000 nerve cell*
> *connections—more than the number of stars in the entire*
> *universe! . . . At any one moment your brain is receiving about*
> *100 million pieces of information which are fed into the nervous*
> *system through the ears, eyes, nose, tongue, and touch receptors*
> *in the skin. One human brain generates more electrical impulses*
> *in a single day than all of the world's telephones put together.*
> —Neurozan Web site, Brain Facts

We are *not* saying that primal emotions like fear, sadness, and anger are inherently unhealthy. They are natural and healthy *temporary responses* that help you to process and integrate difficult, painful, or traumatic experiences. But when these primal emotional responses become chronic emotional states they literally poison your body, distort your perceptions, affect your judgment, and alter your personality over time.

Chronic somatic suppression is an illness. And its healing is necessary for living a healthy, balanced, energy-filled life.

Relax the Body, Calm the Mind, Awaken the Soul

We have to recognize that we are spiritual beings with souls
existing in a spiritual world as well as material beings with bodies
and brains existing in a material world.

—**Sir John Carew Eccles**, Nobel laureate,
Evolution of the Brain, Creation of the Self

Is there any scientific corroboration of the existence of the soul? Perhaps the most convincing evidence to date is three decades of amassed research and personal testimony on the phenomenon of near-death experiences (NDEs). There are thousands of individual case studies of NDEs, and a 1997 survey conducted by *U.S. News & World Report* discovered that over 15 million adult Americans reported having an NDE.

In the altered NDE state they describe an awareness of the self as a soul or spirit, transcending death and the body and existing within a larger spiritual reality. These experiences are perceived as self-evident truths that they often failed to notice while alive. NDE researchers say that NDEs offer compelling evidence not only that there is continued conscious life beyond death, but also that the brain and the mind are not identical, that they exist independently of each other even while they function in cooperation with each other.

Dr. Raymond A. Moody has researched NDEs for the past three decades and has interviewed thousands of individuals who have had such experiences. He has identified eight specific changes that he writes "were present in all the NDEers I have talked to," the combination of which "makes up the luminous serenity present in so many NDEers."

These aftereffects are: loss of the fear of death; heightened awareness of the importance of love; a sense of connection with all things and a feeling that everything in the universe is connected; newfound respect for knowledge and an increased appetite for learning; a new feeling of control in life, connected to a greater sensitivity to and sense of responsibility for the immediate and long-term consequences of their actions; a sense of urgency and concern for the state of the world and for the destructive powers wielded by human beings; increased spiritual development and awareness and a commitment to being a better person; greater energy and enthusiasm for life.

Other aftereffects consistently reported by those who have experienced NDEs include a sense of expanded consciousness, a heightened capacity for feeling, an increased ability to remain calm in stressful circumstances, the certainty of personal survival beyond death, and a profound transformation of character.

How is this NDE data relevant to your energy? The eight aftereffects produced by NDEs indicate a vital shift in consciousness—from the *susto* self, rooted in the socialized personality, to the indigenous self, rooted in the soul. Most spiritual traditions, including shamanism, speak of this vital shift in consciousness as death and rebirth, death and resurrection, being born again, and the like. These same "aftereffects" are produced over time through spiritual disciplines like prayer, meditation, deep relaxation, chant, song, dance, postures, and fasting. Now hundreds of scientific studies have shown that over time, such disciplines consistently produce remarkable healing, rejuvenating, and even life-changing effects in the mind and the body.

In one well-known study, Richard Davidson, at the Laboratory for Affective Neuroscience at the University of Wisconsin at Madison, studied long-term Buddhist meditators. He noticed that their left prefrontal lobe images lit up consistently, both in and out of meditation. "Persistent activity in the left prefrontal lobes indicates positive emotions and good mood," he writes.

In his book *A User's Guide to the Brain*, Dr. John J. Ratey describes some of the biochemical and electrical effects of meditation: "Sympathetic nervous system activity decreases and metabolism slows down. The brain's own electrical activity also changes. Instead of supporting a decentralized storm of signals, a large number of brain neurons fire in a pleasing synchrony."

Dr. Herbert Benson, president of Harvard Medical School's Mind/Body Medical Institute and author of over seventy books, has conducted dozens of studies on the effects of prayer, meditation, and relaxation. He has identified a "relaxation response," which, he writes, "comprises an assortment of physiological changes: a decrease below resting levels in oxygen consumption, heart rate, breathing rate, and muscle tension—plus a decrease in blood pressure in some people and a shift from normal waking brain wave patterns to a pattern in which slower brain waves predominate."

This scientifically measurable "relaxation response" is consistently produced through such "inner disciplines," all of which involve the exclusion of unwanted, intrusive thoughts. "When the relaxation response is elicited," Dr. Benson writes, "the harmful effects of [stress-related] norepinephrine are counteracted. In so doing, we tap into billions of years of healing capacities."

Dr. Haruyama Shigeo of Tokyo University describes in his book *A Great Revolution in the Brain World* how qi gong and meditation trigger the release in the brain of beta-endorphins. These peptide hormones, with a molecular structure similar to morphine, strengthen the immune system and activate human NK (natural killer) cells. NK cells protect the body by attacking tumor cells and diseased cells infected with bacteria, parasites, or viruses.

For several decades researchers like Dr. Benson, Dr. Ratey, and Dr. Shigeo have used modern scientific and medical technologies to study and measure the biophysical and psychological effects of various inner disciplines. Virtually all researchers confirm their positive mind-altering impact, and their therapeutic effects upon a variety of conditions, including anxiety, depression, hypertension, cardiac rhythm irregularities, chronic pain, insomnia, infertility, premenstrual syndrome, cancer and AIDS symptoms, and more.

Not surprisingly, increasing numbers of people in every profession and walk of life, from business and the arts to Olympic and professional athletes to senior citizens and college students, incorporate some form of inner discipline in their daily regimen. And body and mind disciplines that include and enhance somatic awareness, like physical yoga postures, are becoming increasingly popular.

Researchers are also discovering that the power of such disciplines also depends upon the cognitive structure, or belief system, in which they are practiced. Our beliefs are important because, at the most basic level, they affect how we feel, act, and perceive our world and all events in it. And our core beliefs, by skewing our perceptions and influencing our actions, often become self-fulfilling prophecies. The most familiar example of this is the "glass half full"–"glass half empty" dichotomy. Mrs. Glass Half Full looks on "the bright side of things," and her positive perspective tends to make her cheerful, positive, and energetic in the face of challenges. Mr. Glass Half Empty looks on "the dark side," and his negative perspective inclines him toward pessimism, apathy, and depression, even when things are going relatively well.

Still, it is important to note that not all inner disciplines exercise or increase somatic awareness, nor are they always linked to benign beliefs. And the core belief structure underlying any inner discipline will either enhance or diminish its benefits. Some meditation disciplines focus attention in the mind, on a word or sound, or on stopping the usual procession of thoughts, often with minimal somatic awareness involved. Many people practice prayer in a similarly "mental" fashion. Benefits can result from purely mental disciplines, but they will not deepen one's somatic awareness with all of its attendant benefits.

And some inner disciplines are associated with beliefs that are disturbing, at least subliminally if not overtly. Examples of these are prayers to a deity perceived as vengeful, judgmental, angry, or unpredictable; or meditation in a universe that is believed to be random, chaotic, meaningless, threatening, or indifferent to human life. According to a study profiled in *The Journal of Gerontology* (55A, M400–M405), "Patients who believed that God was punishing them, had abandoned them, didn't love them, didn't have the power to help, or felt their church had deserted them, experienced 19% to 28% greater mortality during the 2-year period following hospital discharge."

A famous example of a negative belief structure wreaking health havoc in a life devoted to spiritual disciplines is the great Saint Francis of Assisi. According to the Christian belief structure of his day, Saint Francis believed that it was good to suffer, and saw his body as a stubborn beast under the dominion of the devil to be frequently chastised and ruthlessly "disciplined." He whipped himself frequently with knotted cords, wore painful "hair shirts" that scratched his upper body, slept on the hard earth in all seasons, starved himself through frequent fasting, and threw himself naked into thorny briar bushes whenever he had sexual thoughts and then cast his bleeding body into the salty sea. Despite achieving sainthood, as a result of his beliefs and the actions he took on their basis,

Saint Francis died at the age of forty-six, chronically ill, emaciated, nearly blind, with the worn-out body of an old man.

And we know many determined meditators whose "ignore the pain, forget the body, and keep meditating" philosophy has resulted in irreparably damaged knee joints and ligaments requiring surgery, leaving some virtually handicapped in later years.

> *Gratitude is the affirmation of the goodness in one's life combined*
> *with a recognition that the sources of this goodness lie at least*
> *partially outside of the self.... As a fundamental orientation to life*
> *it lends significance and meaning to relationships, events,*
> *experiences, and ultimately, to life itself.*
> —**Robert A. Emmons, Ph.D.**, professor of psychology
> at the University of California, Davis

Another pioneer researcher on the effects of meditative and relaxation-based practices is cognitive behaviorist Jonathan C. Smith. Smith runs the Chicago Roosevelt University Stress Institute and has extensively studied relaxation-based disciplines (meditation, prayer, yoga, etc.) for many years. His research also shows that such disciplines produce maximum benefits when supported by "positive cognitive structures."

An ideal inner discipline develops somatic awareness within a healthy, positive belief structure that puts one emotionally and existentially at ease. Such a belief structure reveals an ultimately benign, loving universe or Power as the source of all life. It suggests that we are intimately related to and interdependent with this Power. And that we can trust it to provide the energy we need to live a full, meaningful, even joyful life.

Such a belief structure is pointed to by most religions and spiritual traditions, and by current theories in quantum physics. And when we accept, embrace, and live on this basis, we are sustained, energized, and released from a purely *susto*-driven life. When we practice inner disciplines within such a structure, we are able to relax and trust life more deeply. We increasingly experience feelings of peace, trust, gratitude, joy, and love. More and more we come to regard life as a profound and beautiful mystery rather than as an obstacle course in the way of our happiness or survival.

The process of changes described above marks our shift from the *susto* self to the indigenous self, and then to the sustainable self. And the simple four-step process presented below will help you to accomplish this shift.

The Mind/Soul Gateway: Four Steps to a Sustainable Self

You can do the following exercise sitting relaxed but erect in a chair, on a cushion on the floor, or lying on your back with your arms down at your sides.

The Four-Step Shift connects you to the indigenous self that is vibrant, aware, intuitive, and fully open to spirit energy. You enter this gateway through an intentional shift into somatic awareness that begins to integrate mind, body, and spirit. The ability to make this shift in consciousness at will is the foundation skill of a shaman, and the spine of a sustainable self. The Four-Step Shift elicits deep somatic awareness within a positive belief structure that is supported by current scientific knowledge in psychology, neuroscience, ecology, and quantum physics. Combining elements of meditation, contemplative prayer, and deep somatic awareness, it produces noticeable changes in body and mind in moments, and life-changing results over time.

Step One: Stop...Feel...Observe (unplug from the *susto* self)

Step Two: Relax Your Physical/Feeling Circuits (surrender your body into the ocean of spirit energy)

Step Three: Relax Your Mental/Emotional Circuits (surrender your mind and emotions into the ocean of spirit energy)

Step Four: Plug Into the Web of Life (come alive in interdependence)

We recommend that you first practice this method sitting or lying in a quiet comfortable place where you will not be disturbed. Once you have gained relative proficiency in this method, you can apply it effectively almost anywhere in any situation.

Step One: Stop...Feel...Observe (Unplug from the Susto Self)

Do each of these things with full attention. What do you notice? What are you feeling? Tension? Fear? Sadness? Butterflies? Peace? Restlessness? What thoughts or concerns have been driving you? Where is your energy level? Are you tired? Depleted? No matter what you notice, simply continue to feel, relax, and observe with full attention.

In Step One, you unplug from the energy-depleting treadmill of the *susto* self *now*. You may notice an inner calmness. It is the presence of the indigenous self that always lives beneath the distracting chaos of the *susto* self.

Take one minute and try it now.

Step Two: Relax Your Physical/Feeling Circuits (Surrender Your Body into the Ocean of Spirit Energy)

In Step Two you focus full attention on your body's feelings and sensations. This deepens your somatic awareness. If you "listen" to your body in this way, you will feel what it feels, what it needs, whether it is tired, exhausted, stressed, overwhelmed, afraid, hungry, lonely, sad, in love. This kind of listening in somatic awareness releases energy that is bound up in tension and stress. But we must learn to listen in this way.

The body ceaselessly communicates its fluctuating conditions and present needs. But, absorbed in necessary tasks and pressing concerns, we often fail to monitor our energy states and neglect to replenish our depleted reserves. We may even ignore the body's warning signals until they become full-scale alarms.

Take one minute, tune in, and listen to your body now.

Step Three: Relax Your Mental/Emotional Circuits (Surrender Your Mind and Emotions into the Ocean of Spirit Energy)

In Step Three, consciously relax your mind and the physical organ of the brain, and observe and release your thoughts and perceptions. Do your best to notice and let go of them without reacting to any of them, remaining in somatic awareness. Use the physical sensations of relaxation in the body as a calming "anchor" for your attention.

In this step you learn to observe calmly all *susto* thoughts and concerns in relaxed somatic awareness, rather than being driven by them. Each time you calmly notice and release a thought or fear in somatic awareness, you seal a vital energy leak and deepen your connection to your indigenous self.

Take one minute and do this now.

Step Four: Plug into the Web of Life (Come Alive in Interdependence)

In Step Four you complete the shift into the indigenous self and begin the transition to a sustainable self. You do this by contemplating and resting in a positive belief structure that supports the sustainable self. In a deep, restful state of somatic awareness, you surrender as fully as possible into the interdependence that is your true condition. And you feel and receive the spirit energy of life that pours into every cell of your body.

Feel the truth of this interdependence in your give-and-take relationships at home, at work, at the supermarket, and in your countless interactions with others. See your interdependence in all the complex practical, emotional, and survival needs that you cannot fulfill alone, and in all the obligations and demands, challenges, coincidences, and surprises in your life. Recognize it in the fact that what happens in the world—what you see, hear, learn about, and experience, and even things that you aren't consciously aware of—affects your consciousness, your health, your life, and changes you over time.

Recognize it in the fact that, waking and sleeping, from birth until death, a mysterious power called life breathes in you, beats your heart, pumps your blood, and regulates trillions of bodily processes in you in every moment. Feel your mysterious relationship to this power, whether you call it God, Spirit, oxygen, the Universe, the Tao, or the infinite light and energy described by quantum physics.

Sit for a few minutes in deep somatic awareness. Contemplate and *feel* all of this as you surrender into interdependence, breath by breath. Let go and feel the peace of being lived.

When you are ready, get up and re-enter your life. But stay in this surrendered state of somatic awareness for as long as you can, and return to it as often as you can. It will relax, refresh, and energize you. It will enable you to think more clearly and make wiser decisions in your present circumstances and relationships.

This Four-Step Shift, by which you surrender into interdependence, is the key to healthy functioning in every gateway. Practice it for at least five minutes a day, early in the morning if possible. Practice it at random moments in the day. Learn to enter somatic awareness at will, even in the midst of stressful situations, and access the calmness, clarity, and power of your indigenous self.

In the following chapters you will learn to apply the Four-Step Shift to assess, address, and resolve personal issues and problems in the various gateways. As you do this you will begin to experience a noticeable revitalization of your energy.

5

The Breath Gateway: Inspiring Spirit

Oxidation is the source of life. Its lack causes impaired health or disease, its cessation, death.
—**F. M. Eugene Blasse, Ph.D.,** *Oxygen Therapy: Its Foundation, Aim & Results*

Breathing is the key that unlocks the whole catalog of advanced biological function and development. Is it any wonder that it is so central to every aspect of health?
—**Sheldon Saul Hendler, M.D., Ph.D.,** *Oxygen Breakthrough*

Vitamin O! Spirit Energy!

We live literally from breath to breath. Spirit energy streams ceaselessly in and out of us through this gateway, from our first in-breath at birth to our last dying exhalation. Shamans call the breath "the gate that is always open." And whether we know it or not, our energy levels, our health, our quality of life, and the proper functioning of every cell, organ, and process in our body depend upon the quality of our breathing.

Shamans, yogis, and Taoists have long recognized the breath as the primal link between humanity and the ocean of spirit energy that sustains this planet. It is the meal of life all creatures share, from moment to moment. It is a collective communion in interdependence that unites even creatures and plants in a necessary symbiotic life-support system. Plants live on our exhaled carbon dioxide, and we live on their exhaled oxygen.

On the first day at one of my workshops in the Peruvian Amazon jungle, a woman said to me, "I feel like I'm being breathed." She *was* being breathed. The Amazon jungles are the lungs of the planet, producing 20 percent of the vital, invisible food—oxygen—that gives life to the world. Most of us think of solid food as our primary energy source. We fuss and worry about our diet and rarely give breathing a second thought. Yet every breath is a process of reception, digestion, and assimilation of life-energy in its purest form, followed by the elimination of toxic wastes. Breath is our primary food.

Voluminous research has shown that we can fast from solid food for weeks and maintain or even restore optimum vitality and health. But we cannot stop breathing by an act of will for much more than three minutes. Waking and sleeping, we are breathed and lived, continuously. Every breath reveals our utter dependence on a mysterious energy or power. And that animates and sustains trillions of life processes within our own bodies that we cannot control.

Yet while we live in a sea of infinite energy, we decline through shallow breathing the full portion of vitality life offers each of us. A shaman healer will instinctively observe your breathing pattern to determine your current relationship to life and the life force that sustains you. A Western doctor will pay little or no attention to your breathing pattern; his own is likely to be as shallow and inefficient as that of the average Westerner who comes to his office for diagnosis. He may listen to your breathing with a stethoscope to check your lungs, but he will rarely, if ever, prescribe correct breathing methods that would cure many ailments.

Chronic shallow breathing is a common energy leak and the source of much preventable disease. It is a sign of the *susto* self's instinctive recoil from interdependence, a withdrawal from full and trusting participation in life. Shallow breathing is anxiety based, anxiety producing, and energy depleting. Unfortunately, it is the habitual breathing pattern of most human beings, the "sickening habit" of the *susto* self, and the number-one cause of low energy and much illness.

> *Oxygen plays a pivotal role in the proper functioning of the immune system. We can look at oxygen deficiency as the single greatest cause of all diseases.*
> —**Stephen Levine**, molecular biologist and geneticist, and **Paris M. Kidd, Ph.D.**, *Antioxidant Adaptation*

> *Cells undergoing partial oxygen starvation send out tiny panic signals which are collectively felt in the body as a continuous vague sensation of uneasiness, dread or disaster.... People rarely suspect that the constant vague feelings of helplessness, fatigue... uneasiness are symptoms of cellular oxygen deprivation.*
> —*The Townsend Letter for Doctors*

Shallow Breathing

Most of us are unaware that our respiratory systems are chronically constricted. We habitually breathe just enough to get by, drawing in a fraction of the energy that is available to us. Constricted breathing is a direct result of chronic *susto*. It develops in our early years and gradually forms our breathing patterns. The next time you are in a stressful or uncertain situation, notice how your breathing automatically constricts and becomes shallow.

Chronic shallow breathing is constricted *susto* breathing, whose web of causes spans from our early childhood to the present. Most of us were never taught how to relax and release stress consciously, so we tend to retain and accumulate tension and stress unconsciously, even as children. This progressively inhibits and changes our breathing patterns. The ongoing emotional and physical stresses, pains, shocks, and disappointments of life eventually turn most of us into shallow breathers.

Other factors contributing to chronic shallow breathing may include physical illness, polluted environments, a sedentary lifestyle, work environments with unhealthy lighting and stale indoor air, and even the misguided "suck that air into your chest" breathing advice that was standard in American schools and the military for decades.

Shallow breathing under-exercises the respiratory system. It under-oxygenates the blood and the entire body: the organs, muscles, tissues, glands, and cells. It overworks the heart, which expends 15 to 20 percent of its total energy delivering oxygenated blood to the brain. It suffocates the brain, which needs more oxygen than any other organ—20 percent of the body's intake. It weakens the immune system, inhibits countless bodily processes, and leads to illness, premature aging, degeneration, and death. Many catastrophic illnesses have their roots in chronic under-oxygenation caused by chronic shallow breathing.

Through shallow breathing, we suffocate over a lifetime at a glacial pace, breath by breath. And we believe the low-energy, garden-variety illnesses, and more serious afflictions that we experience, and our premature decline into old age and death, are "natural" and "inevitable." But they are neither. Most illnesses, afflictions, and complaints about low energy are unnatural and could be avoided through proper breathing.

Oxygen, our most essential food, fuels trillions of bodily processes per second involving digestion, assimilation, circulation, elimination, hormone secretion, cell rejuvenation, numerous brain functions, and more. All of these processes depend upon properly oxygenated blood and a well-functioning respiratory system. Under-oxygenation leaves toxins in the blood that are then recirculated through the body. Most of us chronically recycle impure, under-oxygenated blood through our bodies day after day, year after year.

> *Cancer has only one prime cause . . . the replacement of normal oxygen respiration of the body's cells by an anaerobic (i.e. oxygen-deficient) cell respiration. . . . Deep breathing techniques which increase oxygen to the cell are the most important factors in living a disease free and energetic life. . . . Where cells get enough oxygen, cancer will not, cannot occur.*
> —**Dr. Otto Warburg**, president, Institute of Cell Physiology, winner of two Nobel Prizes in Medicine (for cancer research)

> *A lack of oxygen (hypoxia) is the prime cause of 1.5 million heart attacks each year.*
> —**Dr. Richard Lippman**, medical researcher

Shallow chest breathing, the most common form of breathing, fills the top of the lung sac yet fails to expand the larger abdominal and stomach area. The stomach requires fresh oxygen to assimilate and digest food and to burn fat more efficiently. Its under-oxygenation means under-assimilation of nutrients from food, which can contribute to overeating. A fully oxygenated system naturally increases our vitality, reduces our appetite, and burns more fat. And as we receive more energy from less food, we tend to eat less.

Chronic shallow breathing also weakens our respiratory system, the body's primary engine of energy intake and toxin elimination. Our lungs and respiratory system are a sophisticated bellows designed to engorge vital life force and expel toxins and waste. Chronic shallow breathing inadequately expands and under-exercises these bellows, causing them to weaken and atrophy over time. This turns many of the lung's millions of microscopic air cells designed to capture and absorb the life force into toxic honeycombs.

Roughly 35,000 pints of toxin-laden blood pour through our lungs daily. These toxins are alchemically transformed by fresh oxygen into carbonic acid (carbon dioxide) and expelled in each outgoing breath. When the lungs operate efficiently, they expel up to two pounds of toxins from the body per day, or up to 70 percent of the body's toxic load. After passing through the lungs, the freshly oxygenated blood circumambulates through the body, distributing life to every organ and cell while gathering new toxins to be cleansed in a next round of breath. Ideally, each inhalation charges the body and mind, via the blood, with spirit energy, or vital life force.

Mouth Breathing versus Nose Breathing

The nose, with its hair screen, its bacilli-fighting glands, and its winding mucous membrane passages, is the body's primary defense against impurities, particles, insects, bacteria, and cold air entering the lungs, the bloodstream, and the body. The nose, besides giving pleasure by conveying delightful aromas like good food and flower scents, is also an odor detector that alerts us to the presence of smoke, gas, toxins, and other harmful substances. The nose is the organ specifically designed by nature to draw oxygen into the body.

The mouth, by comparison, is a broad, open passage offering a virtually unprotected straight shot to the lungs. The mouth swallows air indiscriminately, along with particles, impurities, bacilli, and occasionally insects, funneling it unfiltered and perhaps cold directly into the chest, lungs, and stomach. Animals are nose breathers without exception. The only time you see them mouth breathing is after intense physical exertion, and then only briefly.

Nose breathing is healthy for other reasons. Mouth breathing bypasses and robs the brain of its rightful share of oxygen. Nose breathing directly oxygenates, stimulates, and energizes the brain. Shallow nose breathing, while better than shallow mouth breathing, is still shallow breathing—which brings us to abdominal breathing.

Abdominal Breathing

Deep diaphragmatic breathing stimulates the cleansing of the lymph system by creating a vacuum effect which pulls the lymph through the bloodstream. This increases the rate of toxic elimination by as much as 15 times the normal rate.
—J. W. Shields, M.D., Lymph, lymph glands, and homeostasis
Lymphology, v25, n4, Dec. 1992, p. 147

Abdominal or diaphragmatic breathing is the most natural, efficient, healthy way to breathe. It is how infants breathe before the stresses of life begin to constrict their emotions and their bodies, including their breathing apparatus. But correct abdominal breathing can be relearned with practice and become natural once again.

Full inhalation in relaxed somatic awareness naturally expands our diaphragm, drawing it downward on the in-breath and upward on the out-breath. This brings in more oxygen and expels more carbon dioxide. The fuller expansion and contraction of the diaphragm in deep, abdominal breathing expands and stretches the belly, rib cage, and lower back and massages, stimulates, and improves the functioning of major organs, including the liver, stomach, kidneys, pancreas, intestines, and heart. Deep abdominal breathing also stimulates peristalsis, blood circulation, and the functioning of the lymphatic system, a key component of the immune system.

Yet while abdominal nose breathing is the healthiest form of *regular* breathing, it doesn't *fully* exercise the lungs and respiratory system. And our optimum health and energy require such exercise. Fortunately, the best way to exercise your respiratory system is also the best way to train your body to breathe abdominally.

The Complete Breath: Wake Up and Breathe!

Twenty minutes a day of deep breathing exercises clearly, dramatically escalates athletic performance and is the single most important factor in the effectiveness of all exercise.
                              —U.S. Olympic Training Committee

The brain and the lungs are the only major organs subject to both voluntary and involuntary control. Exercising limited control over both organs can produce extraordinary benefits, dramatically increasing our energy and health. The most beneficial exercise of the lungs is what yogis call "complete breathing."

Complete breathing directly and fully exercises the respiratory system in a way that even vigorous aerobics does not. Aerobics exercises the respiratory system indirectly, and the oxygen drawn in is immediately burned up through physical exertion. But as complete breathing is practiced in stillness, the lungs and respiratory system receive a full workout and the superabundant oxygen drawn in is distributed throughout the body.

Complete breathing raises the shoulders and gently stretches the ribs and the musculature of the chest, the back, and the spine. The full expansion of the lungs, stomach, abdomen, and diaphragm massages, directly and indirectly, most of the body's major organs. The full expansion of the spongy lung sacs allows freshly oxygenated blood to pour through all of the honeycomb air cells, cleansing wastes and toxins that otherwise collect there through chronic shallow breathing. The increased efficiency of the lungs and oxygenation of the blood reduce the heart's workload, improve its functioning, lower blood pressure, and extend a healthy life span. Complete breathing even tones and rejuvenates the skin, which becomes clearer and healthier. It may even reduce wrinkles.

Complete breathing also stimulates and saturates the brain with oxygen, altering your state of consciousness in minutes, uplifting your mood, producing calmness, clarity, and a sense of vitality. Studies show that slow, deep, measured breathing can reduce anxiety and depression and even PMS and menopausal hot flashes! And when the complete breath is done with alternate nostril breathing, it balances the left and right hemispheres of the brain. Complete breathing is the most powerful way to draw the vital life force that shamans call *spirit energy,* yogis call *prana,* and Taoists call *chi* into the body and mind at will.

As the quote by the United States Olympic Training Committee above indicates, twenty minutes of complete breathing a day delivers dramatic benefits, but even five minutes of complete breathing a day provides remarkable health benefits. Within weeks complete breathing will correct long-standing shallow mouth- and chest-breathing habits. As you begin naturally breathing deeper through your nose into your abdomen, you will notice an increase in vitality; improved posture; improved digestion, elimination, and health; and positive changes in your outlook on life that often include an increased sense of confidence and optimism. (It will also give you one of the safest and most enjoyable legal highs available.)

Caution: Complete breathing is *not* hyperventilation, the rapid successive inhalations popular in processes like rebirthing. Hyperventilation is *not* good for you as a regular practice, and doesn't yield the benefits of slow, conscious, measured, complete breathing.

The Complete Breath

Complete breathing, done correctly, yields many benefits. Within minutes it slows the heart rate, lowers blood pressure, relaxes the body, relieves stress and anxiety, and calms and clears the mind. Complete breathing done with deep somatic awareness facilitates a shift into the indigenous self. In this state we commune in body, mind, and spirit with the source of life, and are rejuvenated with an infusion of spirit energy.

When you do the complete breath exercise below, or when you breathe deeply at random moments in the day, remember and *feel* that you are also being breathed. Taste each breath the way you taste water when you're very thirsty. As you breathe in the energy of life, consciously surrender into interdependence and come to rest in your indigenous self.

Preparation

Sit comfortably erect with your feet flat on the floor, or in cross-legged meditation posture. Relax your body and close your eyes. Take one minute and do the Four-Step Shift process. If you've practiced this process daily for a week, one minute—fifteen seconds for each step—should bring you into a state of relaxed somatic awareness.

One Complete Breath Cycle

One cycle of the complete breath is: a full inhalation, lasting eight to twelve seconds, with a prolonged retention; and a full exhalation, lasting eight to twelve seconds, with a prolonged "empty retention." There is no one correct rhythm of breathing in terms of seconds counted for inhalation, exhalation, and retention. The important thing is that your breathing be slow, measured, full, and relaxed.

Both inhale and exhale are comprised of three parts done in one slow, fluid motion. Inhale from bottom to top and fill up the abdomen through the chest. And exhale from top to bottom, emptying the chest down through the abdomen, according to the instructions below.

Complete Breath Instructions

1. Inhale slowly through the nose, breathing into the lower belly and allowing it to expand and swell forward.
2. When the belly is full, continue inhaling so that the middle area of the solar plexus expands and rises. (You will notice that the shoulders also naturally rise and the spine straightens with the breath.)
3. Continue inhaling, allowing the breath to rise into the chest and the upper lungs. Notice how the chest rises and expands with the breath. Inhale to the point of fullness, but not to the point of unpleasant discomfort.

4. Hold the in-breath for eight to twelve seconds. Feel a radiant energy charging your body.

5. Begin exhaling through the nose. Let your chest fall as you release the breath from the top down.

6. When the air is exhaled from the chest, begin to press in the solar plexus and force the air out of it.

7. With the solar plexus emptied, complete the exhale by pressing in the lower stomach and abdomen until all of the air is expelled.

8. Hold the out-breath for eight to twelve seconds.

9. Repeat the entire cycle twelve to twenty-four times. When you have finished, sit quietly for several minutes, feeling the sense of deep relaxation and peace that comes when the body is fully oxygenated in this way.

Suggestions

Practice the complete breath in the morning for at least five minutes, ten minutes, or more if possible. Practice taking complete breaths at random moments in the day. Complete breathing will recharge your energy, calm your emotions, clear your mind, and change your state. It is more refreshing and reliable than a third or fifth cup of coffee at the low-energy time of your day. And it's free!

6

The Water Gateway: Thirsting for Life

The water content of cells participates either directly or indirectly in all biochemical reactions. Denying yourself optimal supplies of water accelerates the aging of the body just as failing to replenish and change oil regularly accelerates the aging of an automobile engine.

—**William D. Holloway, Jr.,** and **Herb Joiner-Bey, N.D.,**
Water: The Foundation of Youth, Health, and Beauty

Shamans have always emphasized the primal relationship with water as a key factor in our energy and health. Our life begins in water, and virtually *as* water. We evolve from conception as an egg to birth as a human being while floating in the amniotic sea of the womb. Our developing fetus, initially 99 percent water, solidifies to 80 percent water at birth. Our liquid nature diminishes with age. By adulthood we are 70 percent water. (This is an average—our brains are 85 percent water, our muscles and tissues are 75 percent water, and our bones are 22 percent water.) Reduced to 50 percent water in our latter years, all our physical and biochemical parts and functions, utterly dependent upon water, are winding down. The increasing brittleness and fragility of old age is a drying-up toward death.

Most of us needlessly hasten our dehydration, unaware that water is a primary nourishment and an essential medicine, the very stuff of life. Through ignorance, negligence, and bad habits, we fail to self-hydrate sufficiently, and decline prematurely into enervation, illness, aging, and death.

So let's take a look at the body's remarkable relationship to, and dependence upon, water for energy, health, and life.

A World of Water Wrapped in Skin

The body is an infinitely complex system of rivers, streams, channels, and tides, from the major arteries and veins to the microscopic water passageways that riddle each cell. This system conducts a ceaseless flow of liquid life that nourishes, cleanses, and sustains every part and function of the body. It delivers water, oxygen, amino acids, proteins, enzymes, and essential compounds created in the central nervous system. It conducts vast amounts of energy and information, nonstop, 24/7, through neurological and biochemical impulses. It regulates temperature. It cleans and sweeps away toxins and wastes from every nook and cranny, delivering them to the proper eliminative organs where they are expelled, via water-based excretions.

Water also cushions our physical structure, dampening the force and wear-and-tear of gravity on our cartilage, joints, and bones. The very strength, solidity, and resilience of our bones and teeth, the hardest, densest matter in us, depend upon their proper hydration. This is true at the most basic building-block level of the body: the cell. Every part of the body is, at a cellular level, water filled, water powered, and water dependent. Every bodily process involves fluids and depends upon regular hydration and replenishment for optimum functioning and longevity. What is drying in us is dying. What has dried is dead. Water is literally life.

Every cell thirsts for water and requires regular daily hydration for health and life, as we do. The cells in our body are dynamic, living water sacs that communicate with one another via water molecules. Each cell is rendered porous by innumerable microscopic filament-like channels, called aquaporins, through which water passes, hydrating, nourishing, cleansing, delivering oxygen, proteins, enzymes, biochemical information, and more, facilitating the harmonious functioning of the entire cellular mass of the body.

The numerous degenerative biochemical processes triggered by under-hydration, or dehydration, occur first at the level of our cells. They are the proverbial canaries in the coal mine. Sufficiently hydrated cells function dynamically, supporting life in the body. Parched cells weaken, wither, and die, accelerating the aging and degeneration process of the body.

William D. Holloway, Jr., and Herb Joiner-Bey, N.D., in their excellent book, *Water: The Foundation of Youth, Health, and Beauty,* list some of the long-term negative effects of chronic cell dehydration, which include:

- Cell structural disintegration.
- Impaired flow of nutrients into the cells due to compromised membrane protein channels.
- Local tissue resistance to endocrine hormones due to faulty integrity and diminished responsiveness of membrane receptors.
- Chronic fatigue due to lack of enzyme catalyzed energy production.
- Free radical damage of cell structures, including DNA, due to reduced free radical scavenging.

- Inadequate repair of nuclear DNA damage due to faulty enzyme repair activity.
- Reduced production of key bioactive compounds, such as hormones, digestive enzymes, neurotransmitters, etc., which can have a devastating impact on all organ systems.

All of the above effects compromise our health, accelerate the aging process, and shorten our life span.

The same "cell panic" that occurs through oxygen deprivation described in Chapter Five, "The Breath Gateway: Inspiring Spirit," also occurs with water deprivation. Under-hydrated, parched cells send the body into water-emergency mode. When this happens, the body begins siphoning water from lesser functions to support greater functions, essentially sacrificing Peter to preserve Paul. These emergency operations can produce a domino effect of negative health consequences, all of which may contribute to *susto*, and *susto*-based ailments.

For example, water may be rerouted from the cartilage and cushioning membranes in the joints, resulting in painful joint conditions and accelerating joint deterioration. This may cause us to stop exercising, to become sedentary, to feel lethargic, which can lead to poor dietary habits, states of anxiety or depression, and other negative consequences. Or water may be rerouted from the gastrointestinal tract to a more urgent location, leaving insufficient water to sustain the protective mucous membranes that protect the stomach from its own digestive acids and juices. This can cause acid stomach, ulcers, and other digestive ailments, which can cause anxiety and stress—*susto*—that can contribute to insomnia, unhealthy eating habits, a weakened immune system, and more. These are two of many possible scenarios that may be caused by chronic under-hydration.

Consider a partial list of bodily fluids that require regular water replenishment for our optimum health and functioning:

- The vitreous, gel-like fluids that fill the central cavity of the eye.
- The tears that clean, moisten, and lubricate the eyes.
- The fluids that lubricate all of the joints, from those in the toes and major limbs to the delicate vertebrae in the spine. This includes the cushioning membranes between or surrounding our joints, the synovial linings, sheaths and tendons, and the cartilage that separates and buffers joints and limbs.
- Urine that expels water-soluble toxins and waste.
- Perspiration that eliminates wastes from the body and regulates temperature.
- The blood that delivers essential nutrients, oxygen, and water to all of the cells and organs of the body, cleanses them of toxins, and delivers these toxins to the proper eliminative organs where they can be expelled from the body.
- All of the fluids in both male and female sexual and reproductive organs and functions.
- The lymph fluids that deliver proteins, fats, and disease-fighting lymphocytes to the blood and flush unhealthy microorganisms and toxic debris from the tissues.
- The central nervous system's cerebrospinal fluids.
- The various digestive and eliminative fluids in the salivary glands, the stomach, the large and small intestines, the liver, pancreas, and colon.
- And there are many more.

Despite our utter dependence upon water for life and its crucial importance for our energy and health, most of us take water for granted. We casually replace it with juice, tea, and artificial "thirst quenchers" that actively leach water, vital nutrients, and essential elements from our bodies. Despite its recent fad status, most people regard water as a poor man's drink and link the quenching of thirst with taste and sweetness, or with high-tech concoctions that allegedly improve on the virtues of water. But habitual ingestion of nonhydrating (and in many cases actively dehydrating) beverages or even high-tech "replenishing" sports drinks (most of them sugar based) in place of water distorts the senses of thirst and satiation while undermining proper hydration. Many people think the water in the artificial beverages they consume meets their daily water requirements. A can of soda is just twelve ounces of water with a few other ingredients thrown in, right? A sports drink with electrolytes, amino acids, vitality herbs, and other healthy additives is superior to a glass of plain old water, right?

Jenny, a twenty-four-year-old computer-software salesperson, drank five or more cups of black tea a day for years, a habit she developed to keep a rigorous study schedule in high school and college. She never drank water, and imagined that the water in her tea was hydrating her system. Her body could take the water in the tea and use it, right? Wrong. She wondered why her urine was always dark yellow. She tended to be sedentary, to eat snack and junk foods, along with her tea, for her afternoon "energy boost," and was always at least thirty pounds overweight. And she had regular headaches and often felt tired, lethargic, and periodically anxious and depressed. She was, by her own admission, a buttoned-down, low-energy, nose-to-the-grindstone computer/office nerd.

When she learned that her tea was not hydrating her body but was in fact dehydrating it, she started drinking eight glasses of clear water a day. Within two weeks, her energy level increased, her urine became clear, and her concentration noticably improved. She soon began cleaning up her diet, eating less snack and junk food, and even started exercising for the first time. Today, years later, she still drinks eight or more glasses of clear water a day, eats a healthy diet, runs three miles a day, meditates, does breathing exercises, and is in the peak of health in mind, body, and spirit. And all who know her marvel at her energetic, juicy, vivacious personality. The simple discipline of drinking sufficient water began a whole new health cycle in her life.

No liquid designed by man can substitute for water, which is essential for energy and health. Other than an occasional fresh-squeezed fruit juice, I have rarely seen shaman don Antonio drink anything but pure uncarbonated water. He consistently declines offers of sodas and artificial beverages when we are in Iquitos. He uses fresh river water in many of his healing rituals and medicinal preparations, and has referred on many occasions to the "spirit of water."

On one of my visits to him I asked him to tell me why he placed such importance on water in his healing rituals and in his life. We sat on his front porch looking out over the river on a hot jungle day. Sweat was pouring down my neck and back. A jug of river water and two glasses sat on a wooden table between us.

"Ahhh, yes, water," he said, "it is a very powerful spirit indeed!" He took a long draught from his glass and smacked his lips. "Water cures thirst," he said simply. "Water gives you your voice, not only physically but spiritually. When you drink water, you are able to speak, to express who you are in the world. Water gives life. The flow of water down your throat nourishes the flow of life that pours through you in each moment, even while you sleep. Without water, your voice, your body, and the earth itself would dry up like dead leaves." Don Antonio took another drink from his glass and continued, "I have heard that in dry places, people live and die by water, and sometimes even kill for water. I have also heard that much of

Shamans see all water as part of one great river of life. Rivers, lakes, and oceans are the most potent reservoirs of living water. When we bathe in them, we absorb all of the vital energies they contain, including the energies of all the living creatures and plants that reside in or come in contact with them, and the energies of the sun, the wind, and the elements of the earth on which they rest. The next time you take a dip or a swim in a local pond, river, or the ocean, do the Four-Step Shift first, enter deep somatic awareness. Then, when you enter the water, consciously feel and absorb its spirit and revitalizing power into your body and mind.

the water on our planet is being contaminated. We must be respectful of water and show gratitude for its many gifts. It is sacred. Remember this with each glass you drink and its spirit will be at work in you."

We live in the most polluted period of human history. Daily, our bodies ingest or absorb hundreds of man-made toxins and chemicals and artificial additives and ingredients from our food, water, air, and our home and work environments.

Flushing these toxins from our body, along with the usual wastes, requires an ample daily intake of pure water. Yet millions of Americans live in chronic states of under-hydration to which they have adapted over time. Like the proverbial frog placed in a pot of cold water heated slowly to a boil, they adapt to the increasingly negative effects of chronic under-hydration, which include diminished energy, stamina, and clarity; increasing toxicity; a weakened immune system; regular ailments and illnesses; and premature decline, aging, and death.

Chronic under-hydration does not single-handedly cause these afflictions, but it triggers biochemical and physical processes and conditions that combine with other factors to make these afflictions virtually inevitable over time. Medical science has established clear and compelling links between chronic under-hydration and the above degenerative conditions. Yet few of us link our own enervation, illnesses, or declining health to our failure to drink sufficient clean water. We look instead for more dramatic external reasons, to circumstances beyond our control, to explain to ourselves the seeming mystery of low energy and poor health. And in our increasingly toxic world, it isn't hard to find plausible explanations.

> *Chronic cellular dehydration painfully and prematurely kills. Its initial outward manifestations have until now been labeled as diseases of unknown origin.*
> —**Dr. F. Batmanghelidj**, pioneer water researcher
> and author of *Your Body's Many Cries for Water*

Most modern industrial city water sources are contaminated with unhealthy additives and toxins like chlorine, fluoride, arsenic, lead, sulfites, nitrates, pesticides, MTBEs, and even radon, a radioactive gas. Yet the availability of high-quality bottled water and water filters in our culture gives us virtually unlimited access to pure water. Still, a third of us drinks only up to three cups of the recommended eight cups of water daily required for our body's basic hydration needs and our optimum health. According to current estimates, roughly half of all Americans are chronically under-hydrated. Meanwhile an estimated 2 billion humans on our planet lack regular access to clean water, while roughly 3 million annually suffer serious illness and death as a direct result of drinking contaminated water.

Water is the only liquid that "cures" chronic under-hydration. Regular, sufficient hydration—ideally eight glasses of water minimum spread out over the day—is one of the best preventative medicines we can take. Sedentary, we lose an average of nine to twelve cups of water per day via sweat, breath, feces, and urine. If we exercise or engage in physical labor, we lose much more. In a basic aerobic workout we lose 1.5 quarts of water. Chronic failure to replenish water loss fully reduces the body to droughtlike conditions, leaving us vulnerable to all of the above-mentioned energy and health consequences.

Chronic under-hydration compromises literally every bodily part and process over time, from the cells, tissues, muscles, and bones to all of the organs, especially the brain, which is 85 percent water. In the short term, under-hydration diminishes our physical energy and our mental clarity and focus, and affects the way we feel and function. Various studies have linked chronic under-hydration to depression, chronic fatigue, fibromyalgia, ulcers, headaches, compromised liver function, urinary infections, constipation, bad breath, and even obesity. (Many people misinterpret thirst as a hunger signal and eat unnecessarily when a glass of water would satisfy.) Chronic under-hydration also thickens the blood and reduces blood volume, causing the heart to work harder and wear out faster.

Unfortunately, many doctors tend to overprescribe medications that use up the body's water for many under-hydration-based ailments, without addressing chronic under-hydration itself. Senior citizens are the most under-hydrated and overmedicated group. They have the weakest sense of thirst and are the most vulnerable to chronic under-hydration and its numerous corollary ailments, which are erroneously considered natural or inevitable side effects of old age.

Common Poor Hydration Habits

Developing healthy hydration habits for an energy-filled, energy-efficient life requires education, intention, and a little discipline. It is very easy to forget to drink water, to put off drinking water, or even, in our soft-drink culture, to drink no water at all. Below are five common dehydrating habits. See how many of them are yours.

1. Not drinking enough water through the day, and/or drinking too much at one sitting for the body to absorb. Drinking large amounts of water once or twice a day doesn't work. We need to drink smaller amounts that will be absorbed, at periodic intervals throughout the day. Hence, the recommended eight glasses of water spaced throughout a day.

2. Drinking only when we are consciously thirsty. Thirst is not an early-warning signal of the body's need for water. It is an alarm. Drinking only when thirst grabs our attention is like breathing only when we start to feel suffocated. By the time we are conscious of thirst, we are already under-hydrated and functioning at less than our optimum. Don't think of drinking as thirst quenching, but as water replenishing.

3. Drinking and stopping when our immediate thirst seems quenched. The standard three to five gulps from a water fountain once or twice a day is a water-starvation diet. The quenching of immediate thirst is not a sign that the body's water needs have been met. Our thirst can feel quenched when our cells are still parched. This is an unreliable measure of the body's water needs.

4. Quenching our thirst with sweetened beverages full of artificial ingredients and chemical additives. These drinks seem to quench our thirst, yet they do not replenish the body's water. The habit of reaching for false thirst-quenchers is at the root of much under-hydration, lowered energy symptoms, and ailments.

5. Drinking dehydrating beverages like coffee, caffeinated tea, or alcohol without drinking sufficient water to cleanse them from our system. Caffeinated drinks are a staple "energy booster" worldwide, and alcohol is a staple social beverage. Both deplete the body's water and trigger negative biochemical processes in various parts and organs of the body. If you drink either beverage on a regular basis, you need to increase your daily water intake to make up for it. Someone who drinks two or more cups of coffee a day needs to drink more water than a non–coffee drinker.

The Soft Drink Epidemic

Many ingredients in sodas and artificial beverages leach essential nutrients and minerals from the body. Excessive consumption of soft drinks in particular is unhealthy, and not only due to the high sugar content. The aluminum in soda cans leaches into the soda itself, becoming an unintended and toxic part of the beverage. (Aluminum is now believed to be a factor in Alzheimer's disease.) The high phosphate content in most sodas lowers the body's serum calcium level. These phosphates trigger excessive calcium loss via the urine, weakening bones and teeth and contributing to bone maladies like osteoporosis, and to impaired calcification in the developing bones of children. Carbonated drinks also cause gastric distension, elevating acid levels in the stomach.

Recent studies have even linked esophagus cancer to excessive consumption of carbonated drinks.

Water Is Alive, but Is It Conscious?

Water is the medium through which biochemicals and neurological impulses communicate information throughout the body. Recent research indicates that water may have the capacity to contain, memorize, and embody energy and information—or consciousness. A remarkable study conducted by Japanese scientist Dr. Masaru Emoto has shed new light on these dynamic properties of water.

In the early 1990s Dr. Emoto, a researcher studying the properties of water, conceived a unique research experiment on a whimsical inspiration. Opening a book, he glanced at a passage that said no two snow crystals are identical. It occurred to him that this should also be true of frozen water crystals. Thus his research project studying frozen water crystals was born.

With the help of an assistant, he first began freezing different kinds of water and photographing the microscopic crystals. He used tap water, lake water, microwaved water, purified water, and even water from the healing pool at Lourdes. He discovered that different kinds of water had different crystal-producing capacities. For instance, he found that chlorinated water and microwaved water consistently lack the capacity to form complete crystals, while water from Lourdes and pure, fresh water consistently formed beautiful crystals. After studying the crystals formed in various types of water, his research took an interesting turn. Emoto and his assistant began exposing water to music before freezing it.

"The results astounded us," he writes in *Hidden Messages in Water*. "Beethoven's Pastoral Symphony, with its bright and clear tones, resulted in beautiful and well-formed crystals. Mozart's 40th Symphony, a graceful prayer to beauty, created crystals that were delicate and elegant. And the crystals formed by exposure to Chopin's étude in E, Op. 10, No. 3, surprised us with their lovely detail. All the water that we exposed the classical music to resulted in well-formed crystals with distinct characteristics. In contrast, the water exposed to violent heavy metal music resulted in fragmented and malformed crystals at best."

Next they began exposing the water to specific words and thoughts, such as "Thank you," "Fool!" and "Love and gratitude," in different languages. Consistently, water exposed to negative, angry, or abusive sentiments produced fragmented, distorted, or malformed crystals, while water exposed to positive or loving sentiments formed exquisitely beautiful crystals. Also, they found that devitalized microwaved water was revitalized after exposure to positive sentiments, fully regaining its crystal-forming capacity. This would come as no surprise to shamans and priests in almost every religion who pray over water for ceremonial and healing uses.

Masaru Emoto's unique experiments demonstrate photographically water's apparent capacity to receive, embody, and express information at a molecular level. He has published the remarkable photographs of these crystals, and the story of his experiments, in a series of books.

So what are the implications of Emoto's experiments for human energy and health? We know that we are water-based creatures down to our very cells. We also know that positive and negative thoughts, feelings, and experiences send corresponding biochemicals coursing through our bodies in the tides of water that ceaselessly flow through us. It follows from Masaru Emoto's discoveries that our thoughts, feelings, and experiences impregnate the water molecules in our bodies with corresponding energy and information patterns. These may be exquisitely beautiful or fragmented and malformed, and both have energetic consequences for our health and well-being.

Also, if positive, loving sentiments heal and revitalize water damaged by negative magnetic fields (as with microwaved water), then they may well heal and revitalize the water in us, and the cellular life in us that has been damaged by toxic thoughts, emotions, and experiences. This is in fact what happens when we pray, meditate, and shift from *susto*-consciousness into states of calmness, peace, joy, gratitude, love. Such healing, revitalizing states of consciousness charge and revitalize the water that flows within us, and thus every water-based cell in our bodies.

But positive thoughts and energy cannot make up for a lack of the basic hydration our bodies require daily. There is no substitute for the simple daily habit of regular, periodic water consumption.

Water Prescription for Greater Energy and Health

The minimum recommended daily water intake for adults is sixty-four ounces. Children need less. It is best to drink many absorbable portions throughout the day. Slowly drinking one eight-ounce glass of water eight times a day is ideal. If you do vigorous manual labor, if you exercise regularly, if you take medications, if you drink coffee or caffeinated tea, if you eat a high-protein diet, or if you live in heated climes, you may need to increase your water intake. If possible, always keep a bottle or glass of water nearby as you work.

You may notice as you drink more water that your energy level increases and your need for "energy stimulants" like coffee, tea, soda, and candy diminishes. Only water drunk daily in sufficient amounts properly hydrates our bodies and our cells. Fulfilling this energy prescription will help you avoid more drastic health prescriptions later on. We hope that this chapter has motivated you to do this.

HYDRATION MEDITATION

We recommend the following water prescription for an energy boost in the low-energy period of the afternoon, instead of an afternoon snack or a soda, coffee, or tea. Pour twelve ounces of pure water into a glass. Sit comfortably and hold it between the palms of your hands. Relax, close your eyes, and notice your energy level, how you feel physically, mentally, and emotionally. Now take three complete breaths and shift into somatic awareness. As you exhale, feel and visualize energy from your heart and solar plexus flowing directly into the glass of water. Also feel and visualize energy pouring out through the palms of both hands into the water. Say a prayer or blessing into the water, silently or aloud. Then drink the glass of water slowly as a meditation. Pause between swallows. And with each swallow, feel that you are taking nourishing, spirit-filled water into your body and mind. Notice the shift in your energy level when you are finished. This water meditation, followed by a brisk walk, makes a marvelous afternoon tonic.

7

The Food Gateway: The Hunger Within

We all know the basic nuts-and-bolts, common-sense dietary
wisdom:

- Eat a balanced diet.
- Eat only when you're hungry.
- Don't overeat.
- Don't starve yourself.
- Eat plenty of live food, such as fresh (organic if possible) fruits
and vegetables.
- Minimize or eliminate junk food and processed (dead) foods.
- Drink eight glasses of pure water (nonchlorinated) per day.

In the last decade alone, nutritionists, doctors, and diet and
health "experts" have written hundreds of books promoting dozens
of conflicting dietary theories and regimes. This should tell us that,
while there may be general principles we can rely on, there is no one
right diet for maintaining optimum energy and health. Most people
change their diet many times over the course of their life.

The problem with many dietary theories is that they address diet separately from its interdependent relationship to other gateways. Diet is not a separate factor to wrestle into shape. It is one of many interdependent energy gateways in a system that is ultimately sustained by spirit energy.

Our health and energy levels depend upon more than the food we eat. *Susto* habits like shallow breathing, under-hydration, not exercising, unhealthy relationships, substance abuse (of cigarettes, alcohol, and drugs), and chronic stress all sabotage our health and vitality. They also influence our dietary habits and diminish our capacity to sufficiently digest and put to good use the food we eat.

Dietary problems do not arise in a vacuum, nor are they exclusively food problems. Many fears, conflicts, and dilemmas are projected into this seemingly simple gateway. Most food problems are symptoms of *susto*, of our disconnection from Source. Most of us, on occasion, use food unconsciously, to suppress stress and painful feelings or as emotional consolation for the pressures and pains of life. When this develops into a chronic habit, food has become another drug that doesn't heal.

Poor eating habits are a primary source of chronic depletion. Our diet must provide the base fuel and building materials our body requires to function and continuously rebuild itself at the level of organs, muscles, blood, bones, and cells. A body can't function effectively or rebuild itself at a cellular level on a diet of fast food, junk food, processed food, or too much or too little food. (Even too much healthy food is still too much.)

The problem is that highly processed foods full of refined sugar, unhealthy preservatives, and artificial ingredients, and laced with pesticides and other toxic chemicals and pollutants have become standard in our culture. Such "dead" foods leach vital elements and essential nutrients (vitamins, enzymes, minerals, and more) from our cells, organs, and bones. They deplete rather than replenish our body, requiring more energy to metabolize than they give to our body. A chronic substandard diet of such processed food contributes to a wide range of ailments, including gum disease, tooth decay, osteoporotic bones, toxic blood, high blood pressure, heart problems, and accelerated cellular death.

You wouldn't put anything but quality gasoline in your automobile, yet many of us feed our body a steady diet of substandard fuel and create a substandard body over time. With a little awareness, effort, and discipline we can increase our diet of spirit energy, our true food and source of vitality, and counteract most of the negative, toxic, energy-depleting forces that we encounter in the world. To do this we must learn the difference between feeding the *susto* self and feeding our sustainable self.

Which Self Are You Feeding?

Sow a thought, reap an action,
Sow an action, reap a habit.
Sow a habit, reap a character.
Sow a character, reap a destiny.
—Anonymous

Your eating actions and habits reflect and reinforce (or feed) either your *susto* self or your sustainable self. And as important as your dietary habits is the self you feed and strengthen *through* them. A *susto* self is the core habit from which all unhealthy habits proceed. And it is a habit that can be changed like any other. And a sustainable self is a habit that can be learned. A sustainable relationship with any energy gateway significantly improves our health and energy levels.

You can adopt healthy dietary habits without any shift in consciousness, through willpower. But controlling your diet on a purely mechanical level may be pruning the branches without healing the roots. A sustainable diet includes healing any aspects of your relationship to food that block your access to the spirit energy it contains. When *susto* drives your relationship to food, *susto* is your daily meal no matter what you eat.

A sustainable self eats efficiently and wisely in order to take in energy, function efficiently, and nourish the ceaseless cellular renovation by which the body continually rebuilds itself. But in *susto*, eating may become an end in itself, a matter of undue concern, or even an obsession. An anxious focus on food fosters imbalanced, unhealthy, or unnatural dietary habits, and is a sign of a life out of balance. Food is not the Source of life, but only one of many vital energy sources upon which we depend for life. Man does not live by bread alone! Breath is food, relationship is food, exercise is food, sunlight is food, sleep is food, meaning is food, love is food, service is food; and spirit energy is the nourishing essence within them all.

In *susto* we may eat automatically, by the clock, without attention, compulsively, obsessively, unconsciously. Or we may eat ideologically, choosing and avoiding certain foods like superstitious cultists or political fanatics following a party line. One young man we know, an adamant vegetarian, described a "nightmare" he'd had in which he'd eaten a hot dog. When asked why this was so disturbing, he said with shrill anxiety, "But I'm a vegetarian! If I ate a hot dog it would betray everything I stand for! I'd be a total hypocrite!"

Healthy food and chronic *susto* is still a lousy diet. Anxious, self-righteous, angry, or obsessive thoughts, attitudes, and beliefs send corresponding chemicals streaming through your body, especially into your stomach and digestive tract. Bottom line: You eat what you think, feel, and believe whether you take a bite or not. Which self are you feeding?

Except when food is literally hard to get, diet becomes a compulsion or an obsession (or an ideology) only when we project our unresolved life issues onto food, or when we lose the somatic intelligence that allows us to eat what and how much food is good for us when we're really hungry. Understanding the underlying emotional and psychological forces and issues that often drive or influence our eating habits allows us to begin to discern and address them.

During my early shamanic apprenticeship, don Antonio prescribed certain dietary restrictions for me: no sugar, salt, alcohol, or grease. For the next six months I followed it diligently, and with anxiety, afraid that if I failed I might "offend the gods" and prove myself unworthy, and that don Antonio might reject me as his apprentice. I lost my excess weight, yet I lacked vitality and I didn't know why. My diet was the healthiest it had ever been. When I returned to the Amazon, don Antonio took one look at me and said, "You look terrible." He told me I was energetically a mess. After an in-depth conversation on the details of my diet and my underlying fears and attitudes, he told me that *susto* had driven my dietary discipline and sucked the energy out of me.

A sustainable self fully opens the energy gateways through vital, balanced, healthy participation—by ingesting energy, conducting it appropriately, and expelling toxins and wastes. In our sustainable self we pay attention to the food we eat, we enjoy it more as we eat it, and we notice its effects on our energy level and consciousness after we eat it. We also monitor things besides hunger that make us reach for food, like boredom, anxiety, loneliness, sadness, or a lack of purpose or meaning. We begin to address and resolve these issues and feelings directly, through somatic awareness and right actions, rather than using food to stuff them down. As we do this, we naturally begin to choose foods that are healthier and higher in energy.

A sustainable self is in touch with its needs and appetites and connects to the flow of spirit energy in somatic awareness. It is less likely to use food to suppress feelings of stress or emptiness, or as emotional consolation for the pressures and pains of life. It eats what is good for it, when it's really hungry, in a natural, healthy, appropriate manner, rather than according to other people's theories.

The Shift: A Sustainable Self, a Balanced Diet

Focusing exclusively on your diet may be the least helpful way to resolve a food problem, disorder, or compulsion. To address imbalances and afflictions in the food gateway, a shaman will inquire about your functioning in the other gateways: Are you conducting spirit energy in the body through regular exercise, through full, proper breathing, through daily work, through contact with nature, through your primary relationships, through meaningful participation in the community? Are you struggling with stressful problems or unresolved issues in these or other gateways? Are you experiencing underlying depression or anxiety (susto)? Are you plagued by a spirit of affliction, a "loss of soul," feelings of restlessness, fear, sorrow, anger, confusion, a sense that something essential is missing in your life?

Most food problems vanish on their own when we dynamically function in the other gateways. When we regularly exercise; spend time in nature; engage in meaningful relationships, work, and service; and practice complete breathing, conscious relaxation, and somatic awareness methods to release stress and shift from our susto self to our indigenous self, we are already nourished and full of spirit energy before we take a bite. Then food is just another form of nourishment, not a substitute for a painful imbalance or an unmet need in another gateway.

But good advice won't heal afflictions that drive unhealthy behavior patterns in the energy gateways. Healing requires healthy actions *and* a change of consciousness.

A Dietary Healing

Laura, an old family friend of my co-author, Doug, worked in the corporate sector in her early twenties, building a future career. Then she got married, had her first child, and quit her job. Less than two years later, she had her second. Now a twenty-six-year-old, full-time mom, she had no career and not much of a social life. And her two very active children needed lots of love and care and, it seemed, all of her energy and attention. Laura no longer had time or energy to do her daily runs, to read a book, or even to sit somewhere by herself and relax.

After the birth of her second baby she began feeling overwhelmed by the demands of motherhood and experienced frequent bouts of depression. As the months passed, her meals became an increasingly important focus of her day. Eating seemed to be the only thing she did for herself. She began snacking frequently between meals. Soon after breakfast she found herself planning lunch and dinner in her mind. On several occasions, while cleaning the kitchen, she found herself holding a snack in her hand that she had, without realizing, taken from the fridge or the cupboard.

Laura realized that she had a serious food problem, with underlying anxiety and depression. She was now more than forty pounds overweight, and still gaining. She wasn't exercising. She wasn't reading. And she was constantly thinking about food.

That was when Laura called Doug. In their in-depth phone conversation, she told him the details mentioned above. Doug asked her if she wanted to do a process over the phone that might be helpful, and Laura agreed. Doug explained the basic principles of the *susto* self and the indigenous self presented in the early chapters of this book. Then he led her through the Four-Step Shift. With no background in meditation, Laura was able to shift into somatic awareness and enter a very calm, peaceful, relaxed state.

Next Doug asked her questions about her participation in several key gateways. (A comprehensive self-examination checklist for each gateway, or *entrada*, is presented in Chapter Seventeen, "Your Personal Prescription to Spirited Energy.") Laura saw how her lack of exercise, her chronic shallow breathing, her never consciously taking time to relax, release stress, and connect in a meaningful way to spirit energy had all contributed to her anxiety, depression, and over-reliance on food. She also recognized that hormonal and chemical imbalances common to postpartum depression might be a factor.

Then Doug and Laura examined her struggle with food and her weight in the light of her stressful situation and her anxiety and depression. Through this process Laura became conscious of the issues underlying her struggle with food, her anxiety, and her depression. She was already aware of feeling overwhelmed by the demands of motherhood, of her frustration at not having time to herself, and of the loneliness of her social isolation. Now she became conscious of intense feelings of loss and grief at having given up her business career; of resentment toward her children, who seemed to need all of her energy and attention; of guilt and fear that her resentment meant she was a "bad mom"; the fear that she was becoming dull and stupid through lack of intellectual and social stimulation; and a feeling of being hopelessly trapped in an unsolvable situation that was consuming her.

Laura also saw her food obsession as an urgent message to herself that she needed nourishment she wasn't getting, and her compulsive eating as a misguided attempt to "feed herself' and provide that missing nourishment. She also saw she was using food to suppress anxiety and despair over issues she did not know how to resolve, and that this made her feel more overwhelmed and trapped.

Laura now understood that her "food issue" wasn't ultimately about food at all. This new awareness of the issues underlying her struggle would enable her to address them more intelligently and effectively.

Laura's solution required developing the somatic awareness and emotional strength to face *and feel all the way through* the painful and disturbing emotions that she was eating unconsciously to avoid, and to access the energy and insights needed to make healthy changes. Our capacity to function effectively as a sustainable self is tested and strengthened by difficult challenges like Laura's. A sustainable self embraces these challenges, and by working through them, it grows stronger and more self-aware.

All of this made sense to Laura. Doug reviewed the Four-Step Shift with her and told her how she could apply it in a simple exercise to address and heal her food issue. This exercise can be applied to almost any issue or compulsion in any gateway.

The purpose of the exercise below is to develop the emotional strength to feel consciously the painful emotions you have been using food (or drugs, or TV, or sex, or any compulsive or obsessive behavior) to suppress or avoid. By consciously feeling in this way, you "digest" the energy and access the information and insight these feelings contain. This is the primary function of somatic awareness, which is the body's instinctive sensory intelligence.

Do this exercise each time you feel the urge to eat when you're not really hungry. You don't have to do it sitting with eyes closed. You can do it almost anywhere at any time, while working, walking, driving, or doing errands. It need not be a continuous focus. Simply enter relaxed somatic awareness and focus your attention on the sensations and emotions in your belly, solar plexus, and chest area. Randomly focus on these false hunger sensations and "digest" them through conscious feeling in somatic awareness.

DIGESTING THE FEELINGS THAT DRIVE OUR COMPULSIONS

Step One: The next time you feel like reaching for food, stop, relax, and shift into somatic awareness. Then consciously feel and assess the sensations you are interpreting as hunger. Within a few moments you will be able to discern if the sensations are genuine hunger or the physical sensations in the belly commonly associated with anxiety, sadness, anger, and other disturbing emotions. If the sensations are those of disturbing emotions and not hunger, recognize that you have been using food to suppress them. And recognize this process as an opportunity to heal an emotional issue and strengthen your sustainable self.

Step Two: Sit quietly for at least five minutes and consciously feel these sensations as a meditation. Breathe in a relaxed, natural manner (not the complete breath). Continue to feel and relax your entire body, noticing and releasing any physical tension, emotions, and thoughts that arise. Don't shift into the mind and think about what you're feeling. Remain in relaxed somatic awareness and observe, feel, and release. If you do this, memories and insights may come spontaneously. They are the information contained in the feelings you have been suppressing or avoiding.

If you are dealing with a food compulsion (or any other compulsion), you may at first feel anxious or even overwhelmed when you consciously focus on these underlying emotions in somatic awareness. Do this somatic meditation for as long as you are able, gradually increasing the time and your emotional strength. If the urge to eat to escape or suppress painful feelings becomes overpowering, it's okay. Give yourself permission to eat without judgment. But eat with relaxed somatic awareness, knowing that progress has been made. Work up to half an hour, then to an hour, then to ninety minutes, and so on. Do this until you can consistently feel all the way through these feelings to genuine hunger. This may take weeks or months, but it will be worth the effort.

If you do this, you will develop new emotional strength and somatic awareness. You will be able to recognize and manage with relative ease emotions that formerly overwhelmed, paralyzed, or drained you. And you will access a remarkable new level of energy.

Laura began doing this exercise after her conversation with Doug. Within two weeks she had made noticeable progress, and felt an increasing sense of hope, confidence, and strength. Within a few weeks she had accessed enough energy and motivation to begin jogging every day in a nearby park. Laura and her husband hired a baby-sitter several afternoons a week so she could have regular breaks and some time for herself. She was now on an upward spiral. In less than six months she had lost all of her excess weight and was in excellent physical condition. She felt calmer, stronger, and happier with her life, herself, and her family. Her crisis proved to be a life-changing catalyst that allowed her to make an important shift into her sustainable self, a process that she continues today.

The next time you feel an urge to eat, do the Four-Step Shift into somatic awareness, and then do the two-step process in the box above. This simple process applies somatic awareness to a specific problem—chronic or compulsive eating—and helps discover its emotional roots and defining pattern. This shift into somatic awareness is the beginning of the solution.

Until we learn and routinely apply this simple shift into somatic awareness, our positive actions will be *susto*-driven to some degree. Instead of addressing the roots of our problems, we will struggle with difficult feelings, behaviors, and situations. This may produce improvement and change, but it won't produce true healing and transformation.

The impulse to stuff (or starve) ourselves in order to suppress emotional pain, or obsess over food for any reason, is always a form of *susto*. But your indigenous self will always tell you, through somatic awareness, if the sensations in your belly and solar plexus are genuine hunger or disturbing emotions like anxiety, loneliness, sadness, or guilt. It will enable you to process painful emotions and access the energy and information they contain. You will naturally develop a sustainable self.

When you function as a sustainable self by conducting spirit energy in all the gateways, dietary decisions don't put a knot in your forehead. You can eat and enjoy your food without concern, and without consulting experts in the field. You'll become your own food guru, as you were always meant to be. Your diet won't be a dogma. A meal will just be a meal. And if you slip into old *susto* habits, you can shift back into your sustainable self with relative ease by taking several complete breaths, going for a brisk walk, connecting to others through meaningful relationship, or by simply feeling through whatever emotions have steered you off course.

Checklist for a Sustainable Approach to Diet

• Don't impose a diet on yourself that doesn't feel good or taste good.
• Savor your food. Studies have shown that when we do savor our food, we tend to eat less, and we absorb more of its nutrients.

• Find ways to use your food consciously as fuel after you eat, for work, exercise, creativity, play, gardening, or any other activity that is meaningful to you.

• Become sensitive to the degree to which you use food to suppress painful feelings, or as a substitute for other unmet needs.

• Before you reach for food, shift into somatic awareness and assess the sensations that you are interpreting as hunger. The sensations in our belly and solar plexus that seem like hunger and trigger us to reach for food are often some form of *susto*, such as anxiety, sadness, loneliness, guilt, etc.

• Make a decision to discover if you are using food for anything other than physical nourishment. Do you use food as a substitute for a lack of fulfillment in other areas of your life, or to suppress painful or disturbing emotions?

• Make a decision to strengthen your sustainable self in the area of diet by using the exercise given in this chapter. Use every problem, issue, or challenge in this area to deepen your connection to your sustainable self.

8

The Exercise Gateway:
Conducting the Power of Life

The physiological effects of physical activity . . . include increased cerebral blood flow and oxygen to the brain; the development of capillaries, which permit collateral circulation; the release of dopamine and serotonin, two essential neurotransmitters that help sustain attention and the ability to concentrate; and the increase of BDFN, which facilitates neuroplasticity—the ability of the brain to continue to grow and change throughout our life span.

—**Gessner Geyer, M.A., Ed.M.**, president of Brainergy, Inc.

Few shamans wake in the morning and go for a brisk jog in the park or lift weights at the gym. But exercise is an integral part of indigenous life. Shamans "hike" in the jungle using a machete to clear foliage, make trails, and cut medicinal plants. They chop and carry firewood. They chop and pound roots and herbs into mash and stir them in boiling pots to make medicines. And they hunt, grow, and gather food. Some of their sacred rituals and ceremonies are also quite aerobic. And all of this "exercise" is done with a kind of reverence, as a dance with life in conscious communion with spirit energy. A shaman knows that if his life is *not* a cooperative dance with spirit energy, he will end up dancing with depletion, sickness, and death.

For modern Westerners, exercise is rarely associated with sacred awareness. Few of us go jogging or to the gym to commune reverently with spirit energy. Many Westerners don't believe in spirit energy. A mysterious, intelligent power shining in every subatomic particle in the universe, animating every cell in our body, keeping us alive from moment to moment? Superstition! Yet they believe in subatomic neutrons, protons, and electrons whirling and revolving within seemingly solid matter; or in cosmic rays, highly charged energy waves and particles rushing through space at the speed of light, bombarding the earth from all directions and penetrating all matter.

But shamans (and yogis and qi gong Taoists) know spirit energy as the power of life itself, and view "exercise" as a form of active communion with that power. Spirit energy *is* the quantum intelligence guiding our cellular and subatomic composition, designing and operating our genetic code, animating with infallible grace the trillions of physical and biochemical processes that sustain us in every second. It is the stream of life flowing through us from birth to death. And when we harness and conduct this energy, it infuses us with a radiant vitality that can heal, regenerate, and awaken new life in us.

Sustainable exercise—exercise done with somatic awareness— may be the most powerful discipline for conducting spirit energy. It literally saturates our body with regenerating life force, from our muscles and bones to our very cells. And it takes our fitness and health to a whole new level.

This chapter will teach you to apply the Four-Step Shift to turn almost any physical activity into a sustainable exercise that deepens your somatic awareness and charges your body with spirit energy. But before we examine exercise and its relationship to spirit energy, *susto,* and a sustainable self, let's take a summary look at what current science tells us about basic exercise and its many benefits.

Scientifically Proven Benefits of Exercise

Scientific studies for decades have unanimously affirmed the positive effects of exercise and its essential role in vitality and health. The most basic exercise, done regularly, delivers an incredible variety of physical, emotional, and psychological benefits, even to those with serious physical, emotional, and psychological afflictions.

Exercise strengthens our muscles, bones, and heart, boosts our immune system, and revitalizes our energy. It releases beta-endorphins, those pain-reducing, mood-regulating neurotransmitters that lift our spirits and even produce temporary euphoria. The general scientific consensus is that exercise improves moods, self-esteem, physical strength and vitality, personal confidence, motivation and productivity, our capacity to handle stress, our sleeping patterns, longevity, and much more.

Hundreds of medical studies on exercise and health show that exercise is a powerful preventative medicine and an effective treatment for heart disease, diabetes, high blood pressure, various forms of cancer, obesity, anxiety, anger, confusion, depression, chronic pain, fatigue, and chronic fatigue syndrome (CFS). Daily exercise can reverse a downward CFS cycle, increase strength, stamina, energy levels, and productive capacity, and reduce the anxiety and depression common to CFS sufferers. And recent studies indicate that exercise may be a useful adjunct in treating alcoholism, schizophrenia, and developmentally disabled individuals.

Exercise and the Brain

New research indicates that [many] kinds of exercise affect the basal ganglia and corpus callosum, sharpening memory and increasing the capacity to master new information. . . . The reason is that the primary motor cortex, basal ganglia, and cerebellum, which coordinate physical movement, also coordinate the movement of thought. . . . Fundamental motions such as walking and running trigger the most deeply ingrained neural firing patterns in these brain regions.

—**Dr. John J. Ratey,** professor of psychiatry at Harvard
Medical School, *A User's Guide to the Brain*

Exercise also improves brain functions and combats physical and mental decline as we age. Many research studies have focused on the anti-aging effects of exercise. It is now widely established that regular exercise, especially aerobics, keeps the body and the brain fitter longer, boosting cellular and molecular brain components, improving problem-solving and overall cognitive skills, and slowing the normal decline of our physical and mental faculties. In one study at the University of Illinois at Urbana–Champaign, a group of sedentary seniors over sixty years old who did forty-five minutes of rapid walking three times a week showed significant improvement in their mental-processing skills and their ability to perform frontal-lobe brain tasks.

Exercise and Depression

Several hundred research studies have explored exercise's effects on depression. The results indicate that regular exercise, as a treatment for mild to moderate depression, is as effective as, and sometimes *more* effective than, individual or group therapy and antidepressant medications. One exercise study had individuals suffering from depression do exercise alone, do medication alone, and do exercise plus medication. The results showed lasting improvements beyond six months in those who had exercised without medication. Antidepressant medications tend to take two to three weeks to "kick in," and their long-term benefits are inconsistent. Exercise has been shown to alleviate depression, often within ten minutes, and to increasingly diminish and even eliminate it over time. It predictably increases physical strength and energy levels, and improves moods and social-functioning skills.

Exercise and Cancer

An overview of twenty-four studies on the effects of exercise on patients suffering from a variety of cancers published in the *Annals of Behavioral Medicine* concluded that regular exercise gave patients relief from pain, nausea, diarrhea, depression, anxiety, and fatigue, markedly improving their emotional, physical, and psychological well-being. Results of over fifty colon-cancer research studies showed that regular exercise reduces by 50 percent one's chances of developing colon cancer. And Canadian cancer researchers have concluded that a thirty-minute brisk daily walk reduces the risk of breast cancer by an average of 30 percent. Nonsmokers and teetotalers who do this basic exercise regime can reduce their cancer risk by up to 70 percent.

A research project studying the relationship between physical fitness and cancer conducted by Chong Do Lee of West Texas A&M University and Steven N. Blair of the Cooper Institute of Dallas studied 25,892 men between the ages of thirty and eighty-seven over a ten-year period. The study showed that men in excellent athletic condition are 55 percent less likely to die of cancer than men in poor athletic condition, while moderately fit men are 38 percent less likely to die of cancer.

Exercise, Metabolism, and the Heart

Aerobic training increases our physical productivity by increasing our muscles' capacity to use oxygen and store glycogen, a polysaccharide our body converts to glucose to meet its energy needs. Exercise in general strengthens and tones bones, muscles, ligaments, and joints. It also increases the body's supply of mitochondria, which facilitate cell metabolism and the conversion of food to usable energy. Increased mitochondria means more energy.

During exercise, the heart dramatically increases the flow of oxygenated, nutrient-rich blood to the active muscles, dilating muscle arteries and opening the smallest capillaries. This "feeds" the muscles and cleanses them of lactic acid and carbon dioxide, increasing their regenerative capacity and their physical strength and functioning. This includes the muscle of the heart.

Sustainable Exercise Defeats *Susto* and Awakens a Sustainable Self

Clearly, exercise is one of the most powerful gateways for increasing vitality and health. Yet many of us choose not to exercise. We ignore the body's essential need to conduct spirit energy through regular physical exertion and grow accustomed to the diminished vitality that results. Millions of Americans live a sedentary lifestyle, and they struggle with chronic low energy, weight problems, high blood pressure, anxiety, depression, and other afflictions that regular exercise has been shown to alleviate. Studies show that over 50 percent of people who take up a new exercise program abandon it within a few months. Common reasons given are: I'm too busy. I don't have the energy. I don't like exercising. I have more important things to do.

A shaman would say the real reason behind all of these reasons is *susto*, which shrinks in fear from full participation with life and passively adapts to chronic states of low energy and poor physical, mental, and emotional health.

Regular exercise is an essential pillar of a sustainable self. Basic exercise infuses our body with spirit energy at a cellular level, positively changing our biochemistry, our emotions, and our consciousness. The natural confidence, vitality, and self-esteem of athletes and the physically fit is a testimony to the benefits of exercise.

Sustainable exercise—exercise done consciously in somatic awareness—produces even greater benefits. It combines all the benefits of physical exertion with those of inner meditative disciplines. The spiritual depth, power, and peace of advanced shamans, yogis, and qi gong masters is a testimony to the benefits of sustainable exercise, which supercharges their bodies and minds with spirit energy and anchors them in their sustainable selves. By consciously exercising in somatic awareness, you anchor a deeper consciousness of spirit energy in your being and your very cells. In sustainable exercise, you are not just exercising your body, you are also exercising a sustainable self.

Which Self We Exercise Makes All the Difference

Two basic premises of sustainable exercise are:

1. Fitness and health begin in the mind and work their way into the body over time.
2. You are not just exercising your body, *you are exercising a self.*

Being a fitness fanatic doesn't automatically translate into vibrant health. Fanaticism of any kind is *susto*-based. Remember, every positive or negative thought or feeling sends corresponding toxic chemicals streaming through our body. When we exercise in a mind-set of negative judgments and self-criticism or push ourselves with an anxious or obsessive focus (whether on body image, weight loss, or muscle gain), we exercise the *susto* self. This diminishes somatic awareness, drives stress and tension deep into our muscles and cells, and saturates our body with toxic chemicals. (Our unproven theory is that anxiety burns muscle, hardens arteries, and generates fat in the brain.)

We are always exercising either our *susto* self or our indigenous or sustainable self. We exercise our sustainable self by shifting into relaxed somatic awareness, consciously trusting life and receiving the spirit energy that is available. When we practice living in this awareness while performing the tasks at hand, it gradually becomes our natural state.

Exercising in this state dramatically increases our ability to function naturally in our sustainable self. So let's consider ways to apply these principles practically to your exercise program.

Six Points for a Sustainable Exercise Plan

1. Get real with yourself. You have to invest energy to get more energy, and exercise offers the number-one guaranteed return on an energy investment. If you're physically able to exercise but unwilling to, your wish for more energy is a passive pipe dream. Something is blocking you, and *susto* is at the root of it. Removing or healing energetic blocks requires a shift into somatic awareness and an honest inquiry into the causes of unhealthy energy-depleting behaviors, such as not exercising. Without this shift and this inquiry you will remain at your current level of energy and health. Acknowledging this is already a healthy shift from denial and confusion to self-honesty. It gives you a greater capacity to choose consciously and wisely, rather than unconsciously in *susto*.

2. Set reasonable exercise goals and get started! Find an exercise you enjoy, that makes you feel alive, and that is doable given your current fitness level and weekly schedule. Begin it within one week and do it regularly for at least one month before assessing results. Many people set their expectations so high they end up feeling disappointed and stop exercising. An exercise regimen shouldn't feel like an open-ended boot camp. If you're out of shape, begin with the scientifically established minimum: half an hour of *any* exercise three to five times a week. But incorporate somatic awareness from the start.

3. Begin each workout by shifting into relaxed somatic awareness. If you've practiced the Four-Step Shift daily for two weeks or more, you've ingrained your neural pathways to shift almost effortlessly from *susto* to relaxed somatic awareness. Shamans and other spiritual practitioners trigger this shift through rituals, meditation, prayer, or through simple, wordless intention. Do what works for you.

4. Return to somatic awareness randomly as you exercise. Exercising in deep somatic awareness magnifies spirit energy in your body and mind and anchors you in the consciousness of a sustainable self. As you exercise, randomly return to this state. Consciously feel the alternating tension and relaxation as you exert yourself. Feel the continual shifting in your balance, rhythm, and movements. Feel the flow of your breathing and the various physical sensations. Feel yourself filled and charged with spirit energy, the power through which "we live, move, and have our being" (Acts 17:28).

5. Visualize and feel yourself as you wish to become. Somatic visualization is a powerful vitality tool. Increasing numbers of professional and amateur athletes now incorporate some form of visualization in their training regimens to improve performance, increase vitality, and sculpt their bodies. As you exercise, see and feel yourself as fit, healthy, and vibrantly alive. See and feel yourself as you wish to become. Somatic visualization releases rejuvenating biochemical processes in your body and anchors a new reality in your body and mind.

6. *Make your exercise a series of enjoyable moments.* Feeling energy through movement and exertion is a primal pleasure. Make this pleasure a primary purpose of your exercise. In *susto,* the reward for exercise is an end result—better fitness and health. Sustainable exercise gives us better end results. But it also rewards us with many pleasurable moments that we find and savor in somatic awareness, which is itself an inherently pleasurable state of consciousness.

A Sustainable Exercise Summary

The ability to shift at will into deep somatic awareness is the basis of self-mastery and the key to a sustainable exercise program. Sustainable exercise is whole-body, somatic meditation and prayer in action. It saturates our body and mind with spirit energy at a cellular level. When we apply the sustainable principles in this chapter to our exercise, we re-create ourselves anew with every workout. And we strengthen our sustainable self.

9

The Nature Gateway:
Plugging into the Matrix of Life

Medicus curat, natura sanat. (The doctor treats, nature heals.)
—Latin proverb

The medicine is not in the pill. Only Spirit heals.
—don Antonio

Nature is a universal sustainable system made of numberless transitional, evolving, interdependent forms and processes. Nature is the force of life, endlessly creating, transforming, disintegrating, recycling, renewing, and healing all things, from cells to galaxies. All things in the living cosmos—atoms, neutrons, protons and electrons, plants, insects, animals and man, planets, stars, suns, nebulae and galaxies, and even the expanding universe itself—are nature's fruits and blossoms.

Nature's "atomic power" draws the ocean tides; coaxes delicate shoots through wintered ground (and even through concrete); churns land, sea, and sky with earthquakes, tornadoes, and hurricanes; animates the countless trillions of creatures swarming our globe; and unifies it in the living, intelligent, interconnected Whole we call Earth.

We are literally made of the earth, of carbon, nitrogen, oxygen, water, and other native elements. And our bodies are designed to return to the earth at death, to decay into elements, to be digested into the soil and recycled as new life. Nature is always alive and in process (even in death), in endless ferment, birthing, blooming, devouring, digesting, disintegrating, recycling, renewing herself, wasting nothing, ever.

We are the highest manifestation of nature's intelligent purpose that we know of, with the greatest access to nature's creative power of any creature we know of. Yet if we are nature's most evolved creatures, we are as enmeshed in nature as every other creature, from our cellular and biological processes to our utter dependence on oxygen, food, sun, and spirit energy. The Mayans believed that our bodies are made from a chunk taken from the earth, and that every chunk leaves a hole we are required to fill with our gifts. But in the larger scheme of nature earth is a minor playground, and we humans are minor players, big fish in a little pond. If we died out tomorrow, nature would go on forever without a backward glance, fulfilling her mysterious, eternal purposes throughout a vast cosmos.

Our most complex and crucial connection to nature is with plants, which for millennia have provided most of our food and medicine, the material for our clothes and dwellings, and the oxygen we breathe. An average of 300 to 400 plants is required to produce the amount of oxygen an average person at rest breathes in an hour: fifty-three liters. For all these reasons, plants are a primary source of our life, and therefore we have a primary relationship with them.

A sustainable self understands and accepts its complex dependence upon nature. Current research shows that the mere sight or

smell of the natural world triggers positive emotional states and energizes our bodies and minds. Five minutes spent lying on your
back in the grass looking at the sky will remind you of nature's
power to reconnect you to your own "true nature," your indigenous
self. When we sit by a babbling brook or the sea, or walk in a forest
or field, nature "entrains" us, draws us into her rhythms, recharges
us with life. Her vital force penetrates and nourishes us through
every sense we possess.

The knowledge that nature heals goes back long before ancient
Rome, when the Latin proverb introducing this chapter was coined.
Modern medicine's technological wizardry will never supplant nature's healing power. Modern scientific research is still "discovering" nature's unparalleled healing powers and slowly, reluctantly,
beginning to bring nature into its healing processes and institutions.
Scientists are even using nature to heal nature!

A remarkable research project by Ilya Raskin of Rutgers
University in New Jersey has found that hazardous wastes can be
cleaned up, economically and ecologically, using plants. The process,
in which plants remove deadly toxins from soil and render them
harmless, is called phyto-remediation; it is called rhizo-filtration
when plants remove toxins from water. The plants, according to
Raskin, are "trained" to live on hazardous wastes and toxins from
the soil instead of their usual diet of nutrients.

Pioneer horticulturist Luther Burbank first demonstrated that
plants can essentially be taught, or coaxed, into making specific
adaptations under human tutelage. Now Raskin's work at Rutgers,
in cooperation with a local company called Phytotech, is charting
significant new innovations in plant-behavior remodeling. Since
1996 they have been experimenting with phyto-remediation and
rhizo-filtration, literally in the field of contamination—in the nuclear wasteland of Chernobyl!

In one rhizo-filtration project, they successfully filtered uranium from Chernobyl's contaminated ponds using sunflowers, at an economical cost of six dollars per gallon. The plant-purified water in this experiment passed EPA standards for use in irrigation and even as drinking water. And in 1998, two other companies, Consolidated Growers and Processors, and the Bast Institute in Ukraine, joined Phytotech in a phyto-remediation experiment in Chernobyl, using hemp plants to draw the toxic waste from the soil. According to Slavik Dushenkov, a head research scientist with Phytotech, "Hemp is proving to be one of the best phyto-remediative plants we have been able to find." Phyto-remediation and rhizo-filtration "technology" (or "tech-nature" might be a better word) holds great promise for the natural removal of toxins from the environment and for the healing of our polluted planet.

But our individual relationship to nature is an important component in our healing and energy revitalization. As we said above, numerous scientific studies have shown that *even the mere sight of nature* has a benign, healing, transforming effect on humans. Below are a few examples.

• In a Michigan study, medical records of prisoners whose cells looked out onto barren courtyard were compared with those of prisoners whose cells overlooked pastoral farmlands. This second group recorded 24 percent fewer sick visits to the prison's medical facilities.

• A similar Pennsylvania study compared medical records of postoperative gallbladder surgery patients over ten years. Patients whose recovery rooms looked out onto a grove of trees consistently recovered faster and required less pain medication than patients whose windows faced a brick wall.

• After St. Michael's Hospital of Texarkana, Texas, created a healing garden, their average patient rehabilitation time fell from six weeks to two to three weeks.

• An environmental study of Chicago's public housing projects conducted by Dr. Bill Sullivan and Dr. Francis Kuo compared two groups of tenants. The first group lived in buildings surrounded by, or had windows looking out onto, green landscapes. The second group lived in apartments surrounded by barren landscapes. Group one had a significantly lower incidence of domestic conflict and violence than group two.

• Environmental psychologist and researcher Dr. Roger Ulrich found that viewing nature *after* stressful events consistently slowed heart rate, lowered blood pressure, relaxed muscle tension, and reduced levels of stress, fear, anger, and aggression in research participants; and that viewing nature *prior to* stressful events consistently lowered subsequent stress reactions.

• Drs. Stephen and Rachel Kaplan, co-authors of *The Experience of Nature,* have spent years studying nature's effects on human beings. Their research echoes the findings of many peers in their field. They've found that contact with natural environments relaxes us, relieves stress, induces positive, healthy physical and emotional states, heightens our awareness and perception, all of which enhance practical functioning, creative thinking, and problem solving.

Our connection to nature is primal, energetic, and spiritual. And plants are more sentient, and our relationship with them is more intimate, than we realize. Shamans have known this for centuries. Even now science contemplates, and struggles to come to terms with, compelling evidence of the remarkable sentient nature of plants.

From the beginning of my apprenticeship, don Antonio emphasized the healing power of nature and spirit, both directly and through the agency of plants. "Remember the plants, and trust the spirits" was one of his favorite sayings. Each of my stays in the jungle healed me on personal levels and deepened my connection to nature and spirit. On many occasions in the course of my apprenticeship, I saw don Antonio facilitate healing in ailing people, myself included, whom Western medicine had failed. He always gave credit for the healings to nature and spirit. I was initially skeptical. But my skepticism soon dissolved in the face of the undeniable evidence that his unorthodox, "natural" methods worked. And as I became attuned to nature and the spirit energy behind nature, I began to understand and experience nature's healing power in a whole new way, from a shaman's perspective. One event that occurred early in my apprenticeship is worth telling.

Shortly after my return from a stay in the jungle with don Antonio, my next-door neighbor, Josie, came over for a cup of tea. Josie had been struggling for years with cycles of depression, anxiety, and fatigue. At times she didn't have the energy to get out of bed. Six months earlier she had confided in me that the antidepressants her doctor had put her on had not helped her. At the time I had recommended that she try St. John's wort, an herbal medicine used to treat anxiety and depression. But I was not yet "attuned" as a shamana. I was still acting as a pharmacist, merely substituting herbal capsules for chemical ones.

Now Josie was back, and still suffering. The herbal medicine hadn't helped. But my continuing work with don Antonio, and the jungle itself, had opened me up to a deeper awareness of spirit energy and the healing process. I was a different person than I had been six months ago. My shift into my own indigenous self had also shifted my perspectives. At times I experienced unusual events and accessed "information" in altered states of consciousness. I now saw Josie's problem as a spiritual condition as well as a biochemical one. I ritually prepared myself to meet with her that morning, shifting my awareness in order to access a deeper level of insight and information. Don Antonio's admonition, "Remember the plants, and trust the spirits," informed my preparations.

Over tea, Josie described her litany of symptoms: depression, anxiety, low energy, and hopelessness. As I listened, a brief image flashed in my mind of spirit doctors leading her out into a grassy field strewn with flowers. Trusting my intuition, I suggested that Josie spend some time in nature each morning, perhaps by doing volunteer gardening in a local retreat center. Josie responded to the idea with enthusiasm, which made me think it was the right "prescription."

Six weeks later she called me excitedly to report a bona fide nature healing. After our conversation she had become a regular volunteer gardener at a local meditation retreat center. Her first task, weeding a huge lavender bed, took six hours. At the end of a day of smelling, touching, breathing, and being surrounded by lavender, connected to the earth and the sun's energizing rays, Josie's anxiety and depression had markedly lifted. (Coincidentally, lavender is used as an herbal remedy for anxiety and depression.) Excited by the shift in her mood and energy, Josie continued volunteering in the garden. She also "went lavender." It became the new color of her clothes and bedroom decor, and the essence of her perfume and her daily herbal baths. She told me she hadn't been depressed or anxious for six weeks, and she credited the lavender/nature connection with her newfound sense of energy and well-being.

Nature had indeed healed her, and I gave nature the credit. But I would soon experience the wisdom of nature, and of plants in particular, in unexpected ways. Shamans have always communicated with plants. Don Antonio said matter-of-factly that he talked with plants, and that they revealed their healing secrets to him. Again, I was skeptical at first, and assumed he must be speaking metaphorically. I couldn't imagine that plants possessed intelligence, let alone an ability to communicate with humans. I had seen don Antonio accomplish remarkable healings using nonconventional methods, usually involving plants in some form, whether ritually or medicinally.

But not long after the healing with Josie, the plant world came alive for me in a whole new way. My then husband, Dean, had been suffering from a recurring painful bleeding-bladder condition. His doctors ran a series of tests that neither revealed its cause nor provided a cure. One night, six months into Dean's medical ordeal, I saw in a dream a vivid green plant, like a miniature pine tree, which I remembered upon awakening in the morning.

That afternoon Dean and I took a Sunday afternoon hike along the coast. As we walked, I saw the identical plant I had seen in my dream growing along the path. Intrigued, I picked one and took it with me. On our way back to the car, Dean's bladder began bleeding again. He was in great physical distress. We hurried home to call the hospital, hoping to arrange an emergency appointment with his urologist.

When we entered the house, Dean sat down on the couch. Before calling the hospital, I went and sat on the bed, still clutching the little plant, and began praying for Dean's condition. Quite spontaneously, with my eyes closed, I saw the image of a pan of red Jell-O setting. It seemed odd. When I finished my prayer, I went into the living room to call the hospital. Dean told me not to bother. He was feeling much better. The bleeding had stopped. The condition never returned.

I later identified the dream plant as horsetail, a time-honored folk herbal remedy used to treat kidney and bladder ailments and to stop bleeding and stimulate wound healing. While I held the horsetail and prayed, the image of red Jell-O setting like coagulating blood had appeared spontaneously in my mind. And in those moments, Dean's bleeding had stopped and his bladder ailment had mysteriously been healed. Was it a coincidence? Or had I tuned into nature and her healing influence using the power of prayer combined with the spirit energy of a medicinal plant? I didn't know what to think.

A more unusual event occurred a few mornings later as I walked along a local nature path near my home in Tennessee Valley. I suddenly had the odd impression that the plants were speaking to me. I shifted my awareness, "tuned in," and began receiving a clear internal flow of information. I could almost have taken dictation. It felt like a communication directed to me, with charming personality, by the different plants I passed by. I paid attention and wrote down what I could remember when I returned home. The following is a partial "transcript" of what the tiny blue forget-me-nots "told" me on my walk that morning on April 27, 1995.

Forget not me, but forget not yourself, your true nature, the place within you that is home. This place reminds you of your life past, of the print on your grandmother's dress, the wallpaper in your old Aunt Bessie's room, of the county fairs of your youth, of walks by the water's edge, of innocence and purity itself. Honor yourself as you do me. Honor your past. Honor the place within your heart that is at times too tender to touch. . . . Behold the delicate nature of your own being. This *is the medicine for the soul-searching weary. We will bring you home to your self. We plants remind you of your true nature. We are not separate from you. You are beautiful and whole, just as we are. You do not know that yet. You think you are deficient. We ask you, are we deficient? Do we need fixing? That we bring you to yourself is the medicine. We plants are a community of beings, just as you are. And we have other specific medicines to share with you.*

I looked around to make sure I wasn't being observed. Then, experimentally, I asked the patch of little blue flowers, "What medicines?"

Pay attention to what you feel when you are around us, they—or at least the words in my head—answered back.

Had these little plants communicated with me telepathically? Was this what don Antonio meant when he said that he and other shamans communicated with plants, and that plants gave him information and revealed their healing powers? The communication, whatever its source, was certainly relevant and helpful to me. At that point my shamanic apprenticeship was leading me on a rapid, at times disorienting journey. Unusual events like Dean's mysterious healing kept me from writing off these "communications" as merely subjective inner dialogues I was having with myself.

In another incident, while on a nature walk, a gingko plant, unfamiliar to me then, distinctly and energetically grabbed my attention. It then revealed its healing properties to me through a direct experience that noticeably shifted my awareness. I was later able to confirm what the plant had revealed to me by identifying a leaf I had plucked and then researching its medicinal uses, which accurately corresponded to my experience. These experiences also seemed to corroborate don Antonio's assertion that plants were sentient beings that communicated with sensitive humans.

I didn't know then that hundreds of experiments on plant consciousness and the relationship between plants and humans had already been done, starting in the 1960s with a man named Cleve Backster. These remarkable experiments were reported in the book *The Secret Life of Plants* by Peter Tompkins and Christopher Bird. It is worth summarizing some of them here, as they support the contentions of shamans regarding the sentient nature of plants and their relationship to humans.

On February 2, 1966, on a whim, Cleve Backster, creator of the standard lie-detector test, the Backster Zone Comparison Test, hooked a polygraph electrode to the leaf of a dracaena cane plant. He then poured water onto its roots to see what, if any, effect the plant might register. Backster, a pioneer in the field of polygraph lie detection, ran a school where he taught police and security agents from around the world how to administer lie-detector tests, but his work with plants, involving hundreds of novel experiments, may be his most innovative contribution.

In that first experiment, the dracaena leaf did register a response. Then the experiment took an unexpected turn. With the plant still hooked up to the polygraph, the idea occurred to Backster to burn the leaf and see what would happen. To his dismay, the moment the image of burning the leaf entered his mind, the plant registered violent agitation on the polygraph. It was, Backster says, as if the plant had read his mind. In hundreds of follow-up experiments, Backster proved that plants are remarkably sentient and sensitive entities that register electrical and emotional responses, akin to those of humans, in a variety of circumstances.

Backster discovered that plants respond to human thoughts, feelings, and intentions at close range. They also apparently bond or form relationships with individual humans, whose thoughts, feelings, and experiences they respond to at great distances. In one experiment, using synchronized clocks and timing key events, Backster found that a plant hooked up to a polygraph displayed readings that coincided, both in time and in intensity, to the inner states of its owner *at distances up to 700 miles*.

In another interesting experiment, Backster had six volunteers draw folded paper strips from a hat. Each of the volunteers was directed to go, at different times, into a room in which there were two plants. One strip of paper instructed the volunteer to go secretly into the room and violently uproot and destroy one of the plants. Not even Backster would know who the "murderer" was. Later, after the plant murder had been committed, each of the six volunteers went into the room one by one, where the surviving plant was hooked up to the polygraph. Only the murderer's entrance triggered a violent "emotional" response in the surviving plant. Backster also found that plants reacted in a consistent fashion when a hostile person, or even a dog, suddenly entered the room.

Equally remarkable is Backster's discovery that plants function as reliable polygraph entities. He found that they consistently responded one way when a nearby person told the truth, and another way when they told a lie. Backster demonstrated this for a journalist who came to interview him for an article in the *Baltimore Sun*. After hooking a philodendron to a galvanometer, Backster was able to distinguish the writer's true and false answers based on the philodendron's reactions. Since then, many respected medical and scientific researchers have reproduced Cleve Backster's plant polygraph experiments and confirmed their conclusions.

Yet plants are only an aspect of the whole of nature whose power connects all things in the web of life. For centuries, indigenous peoples around the world have perceived and honored this web of life, and have also asserted that each created thing and being—insect, plant, animal, man, mountain, river, sea, earth, moon, and sun—is inhabited by a unique and living spirit. As we've seen in previous chapters, current science is confirming much ancient wisdom, rigorously detailing through scientific method innumerable concrete facts that support ancient and indigenous spiritual beliefs.

Cleve Backster's unique polygraph experiments have revealed plants to be living, sentient, and *extremely sensitive entities* capable of empathic, responsive relationships with each other, with animals, and with humans. If plants possess this level of sentient awareness, an interesting question then becomes: What level of awareness might the earth itself possess? One compelling answer to this question is the Gaia hypothesis, now being seriously considered by many respected scientists and thinkers.

The Gaia hypothesis was formulated in the late 1970s by renowned British scientist James Lovelock, who was part of NASA's

Mars Viking spacecraft project. According to Lovelock, Gaia, Earth, is a conscious "entity" composed of countless interdependent species, systems, and processes—chemical, biological, geological—all integrated in a self-sustaining whole. Gaia, besides being sentient, is also endowed with the capacity for self-maintenance, self-healing, and continual evolution. This hypothesis essentially affirms the indigenous view of earth as living mother. But it backs up theory with considerable scientific data from a variety of disciplines. And it brings up the crucial question of man's relationship to the earth. "If Gaia exists," writes Lovelock, "the relationship between her and man, a dominant animal species in the complex living system, and the possibly shifting balance of power between them, are questions of obvious importance." In Lovelock's theory, while plants, animals, and humans have their own conscious life and experience, they both partake of, and are transcended by, Gaia's consciousness.

> *Inherent in this [Gaia theory] is the idea that biosphere, the atmosphere, the lithosphere and the hydrosphere are in some kind of balance—that they maintain a homeostatic condition. This homeostasis is much like the internal maintenance of our own bodies; processes within our body insure a constant temperature, blood pH, electrochemical balance, etc. The inner workings of Gaia, therefore, can be viewed as a study of the physiology of the Earth, where the oceans and rivers are the Earth's blood, the atmosphere is the Earth's lungs, the land is the Earth's bones, and the living organisms are the Earth's senses.*
>
> —**Dr. Sean Chamberlain**, Fullerton College

The question remains whether Gaia is a fact of the cosmos or a figment of man's mythic imagination. The scientific evidence for Gaia is compelling, but not conclusive. The jury, as they say, is still out. Perhaps, like the question of the existence or nonexistence of God, the reality of Gaia will remain elusive to scientific proof, a matter to be resolved through personal faith, or by experience accessed through spiritual intuition.

But we do know scientifically, and we can know experientially, that natures heals and restores our energy. Like shamans, we can all access the spirit energy that streams from nature, from the living, vibrant soul of Gaia, the web of life on earth. We can live as sustainable selves on a sustainable planet, accepting our interdependence with nature, fully receiving her life as our sustenance. If the Gaia hypothesis is true, the earth is not just an enormously complex sustainable system but a global Sustainable Self; just as the universe, the Whole of Nature, may be a Cosmic Sustainable Self.

To see a World in a Grain of Sand,
And a Heaven in a Wild Flower,
Hold Infinity in the palm of your hand
And Eternity in an hour.
    —**William Blake**

It's good to see the big picture. But we must till our own patch of ground to make the greatest use of our "chunk of earth." And the "tilling" that produces the greatest gift we can give to ourselves, to others, and to nature, is the creation of our sustainable self. Below is an exercise you can do to bring in the power of nature, shift into your sustainable self, and access the wisdom and spirit energy that nature abundantly bestows on those who become present to her with feeling awareness.

Nature's Rest

Take ten minutes to lie on your back in the grass looking at the sky. Relax and take a minute to feel the power and vastness of Mother Earth, who is always there beneath you, solidly supporting you.

Rest on her with complete trust, look into the blue sky above, and let go and release all of your tension, cares, and worries. Notice how your mind begins to slow down. Feel the deepening sense of pleasurable relaxation in the body. Notice the sights and sounds of birds, cars, clouds, trees. Notice the smells of the grass or flowers, whatever is there. Notice how your sensory awareness of the earth, the sky, the grass, and nature shift you effortlessly and deeply into your indigenous self.

When ten minutes have passed, sit up and take a look around you. You should feel deeply rested and in a heightened state of awareness. Look around and find a member of the plant kingdom near you—perhaps a grand tree, a patch of wildflowers, or a blooming shrub—that seems to say "Notice me." You've made contact! Pay attention to this particular plant. It wants to communicate with you! Explore its visual appearance, its smell, touch, and taste. Is it delicate or robust to the eye? Fragrant or pungent to the nose? Velvety, smooth, or prickly to the touch? Bitter, sour, or sweet to the tongue?

Next, begin talking to the plant, either out loud or in your heart, about your life's woes and what's bothering you, or about a dilemma or issue you've been struggling with. Ask for some guidance, some personal medicine, from the plant. Say "Do you have some medicine for me?" Don't feel foolish. Shamans do this. Nature is hologramatic. Asking any part of nature is asking the whole of nature! If you ask, and listen in somatic awareness, you will "hear" an answer.

Now lie back down and listen, with your heart, your mind, your body, and your ears. Do this for at least five minutes. Just be still and listen. Guidance will come to you, perhaps as an inner knowing, or a vision, or in words. Each of us has a different way of communicating with Spirit. As don Antonio says, "The plants will tell you what medicine they have for you."

When the plant has finished speaking to you—and it won't necessarily be in words—thank it personally. You've just made a friend. If you approach nature and its spirits with humility and respect, it will respond graciously to you. After all, the plant kingdom has already given us food, medicines, clothing, and shelter. Why wouldn't it speak to your soul and give you guidance or information?

10

The Relationship Gateway:
Energy + Presence = Love

If I told patients to raise their blood levels of immune globulins or killer T cells, no one would know how. But if I can teach them to love themselves and others fully, the same change happens automatically. The truth is: Love heals.

—**Bernie Siegel, M.D.**, *Love, Medicine, and Miracles*

Every living thing is sustained by a current of spirit energy as real, more powerful, and more intelligent than electricity. This current is the presence of life in each of us, and it connects us to one another. It is the power that renews bones and cells and heals illness. It is the consciousness that allows us to feel, perceive, think, and act. It is the divine spark in all creativity, inspiration, and love. It is the secret of shamans, mystics, and saints who have always worked through the medium of spirit energy to accomplish miracles of healing and transformation. And it is available to everyone.

When we access this current of spirit energy in somatic awareness, we come alive as Presence, which is a defining quality of a sustainable self. Shamans know that when we relate from this place of presence, even a wordless glance or smile literally charges others with a healing, revitalizing power. A sustainable self conducts spirit energy in all relationships as presence, compassion, and love.

Hundreds of scientific studies have illumined the importance of maternal love and physical affection in infancy, and show that relationship, or loving attention, is essential for our physical, emotional, and psychological growth and health from infancy through old age. One chilling study of a Dublin home for orphaned children in the early 1900s graphically illustrates the negative consequences of a lack of love and physical nurturing in infancy. In the period of the study, the orphanage took in more than 10,000 infants. Only 45 survived. Other well-known studies tell us the statistical mortality rate in orphanages in the same period for infants under a year old who were adequately fed but emotionally neglected was above 70 percent.

We now know, scientifically, that emotional neglect alone can severely diminish an infant's developmental processes, and that severe emotional neglect in infancy can even cause death. We know the cognitive and neurological functioning of breast-fed infants is consistently superior to that of bottle-fed infants, who receive less physical touch. We know that neglect or abuse in infancy damages key forebrain structures and impairs normal cognitive, perceptual, emotional, and social functioning, and that this can produce serious social and emotional dysfunctions later in life, including antisocial behaviors and a diminished capacity to engage in healthy, loving, emotional and sexual relationships.

We also know, from hundreds of studies on animals and humans, that the positive health benefits of love and physical affection, and the negative health consequences of their lack, are significant at every stage of life. Marriage is not necessary to use "our" society's institution for meeting these and other basic human needs. But the many studies conducted on the relationship between marriage and health show that married people, as opposed to singles, consistently reap the following benefits:

- Diminished anxiety, loneliness, aggression, and depression
- Diminished incidence of alcohol or drug abuse
- Diminished incidence of heart disease
- Diminished risk of cancer
- Diminished risk of hospital death
- Diminished risk of suicide
- Improved immune-system functioning
- Improved outlook on life and general mental health
- Improved relations with others
- More active sex life
- Increased sense of personal mastery, self-acceptance, and self-esteem
- Greater sense of purpose and meaning in life
- Significantly increased life span

But while scientific research and statistics show that marriage is a healthy and beneficial institution overall, it can also be a source of stress, depletion, illness, and even violence. Marriage, eagerly sought and prized by most human beings, isn't equivalent to sustainable relationship. Sustainable relationship cannot come from ceremonies or contracts, but only from which self we consistently choose to be with others. And this isn't limited to human relationships.

The easiest and least complicated form of relationship is the one between humans and their pets. Numerous research studies have shown that relationships, and even short-term interactions with animals, produce demonstrable health benefits in diverse groups of humans, including autistic children, prison inmates, senior citizens, and individuals suffering from various conditions ranging from depression to psychosis to terminal illnesses. Consistent benefits of pet contact confirmed in independent studies include:

- Lessened anxiety and depression
- Lowered blood pressure
- Decreased incidents of hospital visits and illness in general
- Accelerated healing
- Increased social activity
- Increased sense of security
- Increased ability to deal with tragic loss
- Decreased loneliness
- Improved outlook on life
- Improved self-maintenance—taking better care of one's self

The sum of scientific research clearly tells us that healthy relationships are essential for our health and well-being, and that a lack of relationship contributes to stress, anxiety, depression, disease, and premature death. From a shamanic perspective, relationship is food, attention is food, presence is food, and love is food. And relationship always occurs either in the domain of the disconnected *susto* self or in that of the interdependent sustainable self. Now let's take a closer look at these two domains of relationship.

There Are Only Two Kinds of Relationship

Relationship is our inherent condition in the interdependent web of life. But sustainable relationship is the ideal, rather than the general rule. *Susto* tends to be the general rule in relationships for reasons explained in Chapter Two. As most of us didn't get all of our needs met in childhood and as our formative relationship experiences were probably less than ideal at best and wounding or traumatic at worst, most of us, by adulthood, tend to approach relationships unconsciously influenced by old fears and unhealed wounds.

To one degree or another, relationship in *susto* is always a stressful struggle to get one's needs met, a struggle that tends to produce the very results we fear and are trying to prevent. Because *susto* distorts and influences our perceptions, beliefs, and behaviors, it inevitably complicates our relationships with misunderstandings, unrealistic expectations, unhealthy needs, possessiveness, jealousy, fears of betrayal, loss, and abandonment, and more.

Susto is the cause of all the painful struggles, conflicts, and misunderstandings in human relations. It is what ruptures friendships, turns workplaces into psychological war zones, causes half of all marriages to end in divorce, and even causes wars among nations. The basic lesson in every gateway is that *susto* only produces more *susto*. It never produces healthy, lasting solutions; those require a shift in consciousness.

Our modern culture's relationship advice encourages changing behaviors without a shift in consciousness. It tends to view relationships through the skewed lens of conventional romance. And in conventional romance, relationships are unconsciously presumed to be the primary source of spirit energy. This burdens relationships with an impossible demand to fulfill a need that only Spirit can fulfill.

Psychologists have understood this dynamic for decades. Now we have scientific confirmation of the above truths. Using MRI (magnetic resonance imaging) machines and PET (positron-emission tomography) cameras, or PET scans, neurobiologists have monitored dopamine receptors in the brain. They have discovered which chemicals are released into the body in various kinds of love-emotion and which areas of the brain "light up" under their influence.

Neurobiological science has discovered that intense romantic love triggers the release of two potent neurotransmitters, norepinephrine, an adrenaline stimulant that diminishes appetite and reduces the need for sleep, and dopamine, which induces pleasure and alleviates depression and anxiety. The emotional and biochemical effects of both of these neurotransmitters bear uncanny similarities to stimulants like methamphetamine, cocaine, and ecstasy. Studies on these biochemical effects and the corresponding psychological effects of romantic love by various neurobiologists and psychologists have independently reached the same startling conclusion: Romantic love is uncannily similar to drug addiction.

Anthropologist Helen Fisher of Rutgers University, neuroscientist Lucy Brown of Albert Einstein Medical College, and psychologist Arthur Aron of the State University of New York studied the emotional, behavioral, and biochemical effects of romantic love on seventeen love-struck volunteers. Through in-depth interviews and questionnaires and by monitoring the subjects' brains on MRI machines, they corroborated the obsessive and addictive nature of romantic intoxication, which is dominated by the effects of dopamine.

"We found specific activity in regions of the right caudate nucleus and right ventral tegmental area," says Lucy Brown. "These brain areas are rich in dopamine and are part of the brain's motivation and reward system. Elevated levels of central dopamine produce energy, focused attention on novel stimuli, motivation to win a reward and feelings of elation—some of the core feelings of romantic love. Activity in other regions changed also, including one that another imaging study has shown to become active when people eat chocolate."

Helen Fisher also emphasizes the obsessive and addictive nature of romantic love. "One of the main traits of romantic love is that you can't stop thinking about the person that you're in love with; it is obsessive," she says. "Romantic love is really a need. It is a craving for emotional unity with another human being."

As the high-intensity romantic phase of love eventually subsides, these intoxicating druglike effects diminish. Then other hormones like vasopressin and oxytocin (called the "cuddle hormone") kick in to facilitate the deeper emotional bonding that characterizes mature love. These hormones, which diminish anxiety and depression and alleviate stress, account for many of the health benefits of healthy love. Biochemically, romance is a potent, potentially addictive legal high. And most people are ever eager for a fix. Yet many people become literally addicted to the romantic high, and obsessive relationships and short-term serial relationships are a modern form of addiction. A burgeoning twelve-step movement called Sex and Love Addicts Anonymous has sprung up in the West to address the addictive nature of romantic and sexual relationships.

But romance, like marriage, isn't equivalent to sustainable relationship, or even love. Sustainable relationship is giving and receiving spirit energy as kindness, presence, or love *without expectation, possessiveness, jealousy, or attachment*. Romantic love's notorious shadow is often entangled with these *susto* qualities, and its irrational behaviors and crimes of passion fill the annals of literature and police records around the world.

Sustainable relationship, by contrast, has no shadow side. (Though *susto* may rear its dysfunctional head in any relationship.) It is always wholly positive and healing. It is the basis of all love but not equivalent to any form of love. It is the current of spirit energy that connects all living creatures to Source and to each other. It blossoms whenever *susto* disappears and we make direct contact with another. And it restores us in a moment to our sustainable self.

As in every gateway, the key to mastery lies in this shift into our sustainable self via a radical shift in perspective, followed by disciplined adherence to sustainable principles. This is true for sustainable relationships. A sustainable self does not view relationships as sources of happiness or solutions to unhappiness. It views them as opportunities to magnify spirit energy, or love, through spiritual contact with others. When we relate to others through the current or presence of spirit energy that connects us to each other, we stimulate this sustainable frequency in them, as one tuning fork vibrating a certain note causes another to vibrate in harmony. Presence is the essence of relationship. And shamans know that when we become fully present with others, spirit energy is transmitted and extraordinary things become possible.

Relationship, from Atoms to Infinity

Quantum physics' chaos theory tells us everything in the universe is connected and interdependent. Atoms, neutrons, protons and electrons, individuals, families, neighborhoods and nations, planets, suns, stars and galaxies—all form an infinitely complex web of relationships. A famous hypothesis illustrating this principle of universal interdependence states: "If a butterfly flaps its wings in China, the entire universe is affected." Scientists tell us that if we had instruments sensitive enough, we could measure the effect of that butterfly's wings in San Francisco. If chaos theory is correct, the same flap would also register on a planet in some far galaxy.

What, then, of the interconnection among living, feeling, thinking creatures? We saw from studies on the power of prayer in the healing process that our thoughts, feelings, and attention have a verifiable impact on others. Most of us have experienced "coincidences" where we were thinking about someone, or dreamed about them, and they called us shortly after, or we bumped into them unexpectedly. What is this link that connects us to others over distances, that results in such "coincidences"? What forms of invisible contact do we have with others that we are unaware of?

We recommend a very simple exercise to test this invisible link, an experiment in interdependence. Sit down in a quiet place and enter deep somatic awareness using the Four-Step Shift. Spend fifteen minutes focusing intently on someone you know. See him, or her, in your mind's eye, feel his personality and his presence, and silently say his name. Do this with a very intense focus. When you are finished, call him up (if he hasn't already called you) and ask if he was thinking of you.

The truth of interdependence, long known by shamans, yogis, and mystics, has been affirmed in the last three decades in an unexpected new field of inquiry. A consistent assertion appearing in the reports of thousands of NDEers (near-death experiencers) is that everything is connected and that our simplest interactions with others ripple out to affect hundreds of lives. And virtually all NDEers affirm from personal experience one fundamental purpose of human life: We are here to love others.

A sustainable self lives in an interdependent universe in which relationship is the condition of life. And it lives on the basis of the following principles:

• Which self we are being in any moment or situation is a matter of choice and awareness.
• Our thoughts and actions send corresponding waves of energy out into the world and into our own body and mind.
• Energy is exchanged in all of our contacts with others.
• All expressions of energy are contagious, all contact with others is potentially initiatory, and we transmit to others and the world our anger, fear, sorrow, joy, peace, or love.
• A sustainable self, connected to Source within, does not view

relationships as sources of happiness or solutions to unhappiness, but as opportunities to conduct spirit energy as presence, compassion, or love.

Shamans, mystics, and healers have long known and applied these insights for the benefit of others. My first encounter with the Amazon jungle shaman in the hut changed my life. This shaman's intense presence drew me into an altered state, and initiated a process of healing and transformation. But this power is available not only to shamans and mystics. It is an essential quality of every sustainable self. Anyone can access it.

In *Everyday Enlightenment*, Dan Millman writes of a woman named Cheryl who told him after a lecture how a smile saved her life. Deep in depression, Cheryl had made two previous suicide attempts. One day she decided to make her third attempt. "I didn't believe anyone cared whether I lived or died, so I didn't care either," she said. As she walked home determined to end her life, she saw a man approaching from the opposite direction. She looked at him as they passed each other, and he smiled. Something in his smile struck her. It inexplicably changed her state. She kept thinking about it. "It was something I wanted to hold on to for a while," she said. "So I didn't kill myself that day, or the next. Then I decided to stick around and get some help. Things are better now. I have a boyfriend I love a lot, and a job I like." Something was transmitted in that smile that changed and perhaps saved a human life.

Doug Childers, in *Divine Interventions*, written with Dan Millman, tells how he was walking home late one night in San Francisco when two muggers came for him out of a doorway. The man nearest to him, dressed in black with a knit cap pulled low over his forehead, moved toward Doug with a metal pipe raised above his head to strike. Inexplicably, Doug's state of consciousness shifted. He not only felt no fear, he felt an exhilarating joy. Before the man could strike, Doug looked into his eyes with a big smile and said, "Hey! How are you?" The man froze with a bewildered look, his pipe still raised. Doug looked into the eyes of the second man and said cheerfully, "How are you doing?" The second man also froze, looking very puzzled. Doug continued walking. Moments later he heard the two men running down the street—in the opposite direction.

These events demonstrate the power of relationship via the mysterious current of spirit energy that connects us all. In my experience with the shaman, it changed the course of my life and my career. In Cheryl's case it may have prevented a suicide and turned a life around. In Doug's case it stopped a mugging, and perhaps changed three lives. If you examine your life, you will probably be able to recall incidents where your sustainable self—or your *susto* self—created corresponding effects or reactions in others, for good or for ill. The purpose of this chapter, and this book, is to help you consistently choose which self you will be and the impact you have on others.

A *susto* self can only transmit *susto*. A sustainable self always transmits a living current of spirit energy that produces healthy relationship. And as the above stories show, it can also produce unpredictable and life-changing results. This is the "secret power" in the spell cast by shamans, mystics, and saints, and it is available to ordinary human beings who, by accident or by choice, make the shift into their sustainable selves.

Two Sustainable Relationship Exercises

The following simple exercise, done with a partner, will shift you into a surprisingly deep state of shared somatic awareness, or sustainable relationship.

Exercise One

1. Put on music that you find emotionally or spiritually uplifting.
2. Sit facing your partner with your knees close together or touching. You can sit in two chairs, or on pillows on the floor. If you are doing this exercise with an intimate partner, you can sit on the floor with your legs wrapped around each other's waists.
3. Sit for one minute with eyes closed, take several deep breaths, and enter somatic awareness.
4. Now, looking into your partner's eyes, lightly touch hands at the outside of the knees. Slowly bring them up together in a wide arc till your hands are raised above your heads, still touching. Then slowly bring them down again in the reverse arc till they are down near the knees again. For the next ten minutes, simply raise and lower your hands and be present to your breath, to the sensations in your body, to any thoughts, feelings, or emotions that arise.
5. As you do this, be present to your breath, to the sensations in your body, to any thoughts, feelings, or emotions that arise. But also remain fully present to your partner. Feel the presence of the soul shining through his or her eyes, meeting yours.

The next exercise can be done almost anywhere with anyone. It will allow you to explore the effects of your own sustainable self on others in a variety of situations. You can choose a situation in advance for this exercise, or try it spontaneously. Either way is effective. Try it at your next business meeting, party, or lunch date, or in any random encounter with a friend, an acquaintance, or even a stranger. The other person will not know you are doing this exercise, although they may sense something different about you. It is your private experiment, a chance to notice what occurs in your relations with others when you consciously relate from your sustainable self.

Exercise Two

In the presence of another person, use the somatic awareness method to shift silently into your sustainable self. Relate to the other person in this state, as a kind of relational meditation. As with the first exercise above, be present to your breath, to the sensations in your body, to any thoughts, feelings, or emotions that arise. Relax, feel, and release any fear or awkwardness that arises in you. But also remain fully present to the other person. Feel the presence of the other person's soul shining through his or her eyes, meeting yours. As you do this, simply relate to the other person in a natural manner. And notice the quality of the conversation, the connection that occurs.

This method is very effective in moments of stressful relationship, awkwardness, conflicts, or misunderstanding. Try this in different circumstances and with different people. Eventually, this will become a natural part of the way you relate to others, and your relationships—and you—will shift and deepen as a result.

The Most Important Relationship of All

You are the *only* person with whom you will spend every breath and heartbeat of your life. Which self you will spend that kind of time with, what sort of company you will be for you, is a matter of choice in countless moments and situations over time.

When Abraham Lincoln said, "After forty, every man is responsible for his face," he was referring to our final responsibility for the self we become. In our early years, who we are very much depends on how we are treated in infancy and childhood. But after adolescence, and especially from adulthood on, how we treat ourselves through our thoughts, our moods, our attitudes, and our habits in the various *entradas* are the crucial factors that determine who we are. In this way, our relationship to our self determines our relationships with others.

It's not just a good idea to "love thy neighbor as thyself." Emotionally, psychologically, and spiritually, it's all we're capable of doing. And when we have a sustainable relationship with our self, our other relationships will gradually fall in line. And we will begin to experience a natural magnetic pull into what we call Reciprocity.

THE NATURE OF NATURE IS LOVE

One day, during one of my visits with don Antonio, he came to me and said he wanted to show me "something special." As we went deeper into the jungle, I felt the shift of consciousness that always happened inside me. My mind quieted down, my body grew more relaxed and grounded, and I felt soothed and calmed. It was as though the jungle quietly absorbed from my being all that was nonessential and restored me to my indigenous self.

We came upon a little jungle clearing and don Antonio pointed to a gigantic vine-covered tree at least eight stories tall. "Do you see how tightly that vine has wrapped around that big tree?" he asked. "This is the *estrangulador* vine. It is the spirit of the jungle, the spirit of love." Indeed, the vine was so tightly wrapped around the tree it seemed fused into its trunk. I couldn't see a clear demarcation between the two. "The *estrangulador* vine loves this tree so much and hugs it so tightly that the two become one. The jungle is this way. It wraps around you and becomes one with you. The energy of the jungle is the energy of love! The medicine of the jungle is love."

11

The Altruism Gateway:
Sustainable Reciprocity

When you make your transition you are asked two things: How much love you have been able to give and receive, and how much service you have rendered. And you will know every consequence of every deed, every thought, and every word you have ever uttered. And that is, symbolically speaking, going through hell, when you see how many chances you have missed. But you will also see how a nice act of kindness has touched hundreds of lives that you're totally unaware of.

—Elisabeth Kubler-Ross, from the *Graceful Passages* CD

Altruism behaves like a miracle drug, and a strange one at that. It has beneficial effects on the person doing the helping—the helper's high; it benefits the person to whom the help is directed; and it can stimulate healthy responses in persons at a distance who may view it only obliquely.

—Dr. Larry Dossey, *Meaning & Medicine*

In previous chapters we've seen how energy solutions and "upgrades" require practical action and a change in consciousness—a shift into our sustainable self. Our progressive shift into our sustainable self deepens our awareness of our interdependence and our sense of connectedness to others, until at some point we feel a new impulse stirring in us—a higher call to altruistic action.

Whether subtle, as a loving look into the eyes of a suffering person, or dramatic, as a stranger rushing into a burning house to save a child, altruism is the highest expression of spirit energy in human beings. Altruism springs naturally from empathy, and also awakens, opening hidden reserves of spirit energy within that we can't access in any other way. To understand the effects of altruism, think of the extraordinary physical stamina, spiritual will, and power it released in the outwardly frail Mahatma Gandhi and Mother Teresa.

Altruism is often seen as something that yields future personal benefit—good karma, peace of mind, a reward in heaven. But many scientific studies show that altruistic action bestows immediate and long-term energy and health benefits upon the giver and the receiver, and even upon those who merely witness an altruistic action. But it yields the greatest benefits to the giver, proving the adage that "it is better to give than to receive." The benefits of altruistic or "selfless" action, from a shamanic perspective, come from the fact that in such actions the *susto* self is released and the sustainable self is awakened. For this reason we call altruistic action sustainable reciprocity.

Author Alan Luks, who co-authored *The Healing Power of Doing Good*, is the executive director of New York's Institute for the Advancement of Health, which gathers and makes available the increasing scientific data on the mind-body connection. Luks designed a seventeen-question survey about the effects and aftereffects people experienced when they performed altruistic acts or gestures of kindness. There were 3,296 volunteers from over 20 organizations around the United States who completed and returned the survey.

The results showed a consistent pattern of positive effects in those who acted altruistically, providing compelling evidence that altruistic behavior yields significant health benefits. The most common effect of altruism on the helper is what Luks has termed the "helper's high," a rush of positive feelings and emotions that indicates the release of endorphins, with all of their attendant benefits. These altruistic side effects include reduced stress; improved immune-system functioning; a sense of joy, peace, and well-being; and even relief from physical and emotional pain. These effects tend to last long after the helping encounter, and they recur whenever the encounter is recalled. They also increase with the frequency of altruistic behavior. And those who consistently help others regularly experience this helper's high and its healing and uplifting aftereffects.

"Helping," says Luks, "contributes to the maintenance of good health, and it can diminish the effect of diseases and disorders both serious and minor, psychological and physical." Interestingly, Luks found that helper's high and its positive effects were the strongest when we help strangers.

Various studies have shown that acts of altruism promote quicker recovery from surgery and help to alleviate a variety of health conditions, including insomnia, overeating, obesity, colds, flu, migraines, acid stomach, depression, ulcers, anxiety, arthritis, lupus, asthma, and cancer. A ten-year study of 2,700 men in Michigan found that those who engaged in regular volunteer work had death rates 2½ times lower than those who didn't. In other words, altruism prolongs our lives. Studies have also shown that regular acts of altruism not only improve one's health, but also transform one's personality over time.

A well-known Harvard research study conducted by psychology professor David McClelland found that students who merely witnessed altruistic action, such as a film of Mother Teresa ministering to the sick in Calcutta, experienced a boost in their immune systems. This boost was registered as an increase in immunoglobulin, the antibodies that fight infection and illness, in the saliva. McClelland found that the greatest immune-system boost occurred in those students with the strongest altruistic impulses, those who most wanted to help others without thought of personal gain.

McClelland and other researchers have shown that the positive relationships we establish through altruistic service are inherently beneficial to our immune system. McClelland identifies one key characteristic that we develop through altruistic bonds as "affiliative trust." And his research shows that the greater our level of affiliative trust, the stronger our immune system. He says, "We have preliminary evidence in a longitudinal study that people who are high in affiliative trust show fewer instances of major illnesses nine years after the assessment."

But perhaps the most compelling evidence of the life-transforming effects of altruism are demonstrated in the global phenomenon of Alcoholics Anonymous, the most effective, successful treatment for addiction yet discovered. In the last seven decades, AA has helped tens of millions of individuals around the world overcome every kind of debilitating physical, emotional, and psychological addiction. And a root principle of AA is that we heal by helping others. Bill Wilson, AA's founder, understood the principle of sustainable reciprocity. And he employed it as a key component in the process of helping addicts recover or rediscover healthy selves—along with the help of "a higher power," or Source. In AA, each new member has a sponsor, an altruistic mentor who supports him or her in the recovery process.

These AA sponsors learn that helping others accelerates their own healing. They apply the principles of sustainable reciprocity: When we do good to others, we do good to ourselves. And the good we do goes out into the world and returns to us in ways we cannot foresee. The first AA meeting, with only two men, was held in 1935. Within four years it had spread throughout the United States and had helped 100,000 alcoholics stop drinking. The success of AA is a testament to the power of sustainable reciprocity.

By expressing this altruistic part of our nature, we are healed of the separative self-absorption of the *susto* self, which literally is a kind of self-destructive addiction. Conversely, *not* to express this part of ourselves is a default whose cost is the "pain of unfulfilled life." And this default robs the world of gifts that were meant to come through us. Sigmund Freud, Carl Jung, Ernest Becker, and other pioneers of psychology point to this unfulfilled life as the source of much neuroses, mental illness, and self-destructive or addictive behaviors.

The essence of sustainable reciprocity is compassionate action. But we don't have to feel compassion before we take action. Altruism *awakens* compassion. It allows us to experience an uncommon depth in our self, and in others. And the good we do returns to us—immediately, as science now shows, and also in the future in surprising ways.

Susto versus Altruism

A large portion of social science research is based on the assumption that people don't behave out of any motivation except their own self-interest. We are in fact legitimating another kind of motivation. Our work represents a bona fide contribution to research and literature on pro/social and altruistic behavior. It also points to the potency of individuals. Individuals do make a difference. We are not entirely the pawns of social structures, even when they are diabolical. It is important to communicate that individuals did make choices.

—**Pearl Oliner**, co-founder of the Altruistic Personality Project (which studied more than 500 ordinary individuals who either risked or refused to risk their lives to help persecuted Jews under Nazi occupation)

Moral courage is not the exclusive province of extraordinary people—heroes and saints. It is available to anyone who lives his or her life routinely in relationships of care and concern for other people's welfare and for diverse groups of people.
—**Samuel Oliner,** co-founder of the Altruistic Personality Project

Clearly, altruism yields both immediate and long-term personal health and energy benefits. *And it feels good.* So why isn't altruism standard operating procedure? Sometimes it is risky to the point of death, as with those who helped Jews under Nazi occupation, who rescue strangers from burning buildings, or soldiers who help their wounded comrades under fire.

But also, altruism seems idealistic and unrealistic to the *susto* self in its myopic preoccupation with personal safety, benefits, needs, and goals. When time is money, energy seems scarce, and we're struggling to get our own needs met, altruism is a stretch that seems to require more energy than we have to give. And yet the very stretch that altruism requires would, if we made it, open up whole new reserves of energy within us.

In *susto*, we tend to move through life looking out mostly for number one (and immediate family). We give *in order to* receive as a general rule, or we may try to get as much as we can while giving as little as we can. Or we may even act fairly by honoring the basic principle of reciprocity. But mere reciprocity still limits our access to spirit energy; it is still *susto* consciousness.

As our shift into our sustainable self deepens, our energy, our awareness, and our sense of connectedness to others increases. And at a certain point, our cup runneth over in altruism, in kind or helpful acts. We have entered the higher energy circuit of sustainable reciprocity. Here we express a healthy, empathic relationship with the whole in all its parts. In our abundant vitality, our cup of life *must* spill over in altruistic action. To access higher levels of spirit energy it must now be given away, because we only get as much as we give away. As we do this, the self-concerns of *susto* are consumed in the spirit of sustainable reciprocity. And this must happen individually in great numbers before it can happen collectively. Unfortunately, the collective is in the fierce grip of *susto,* and encourages it as a lifestyle.

Modern *susto* consumer culture embraces altruism in theory, yet rejects it in practice. By valuing short-term personal benefit over a larger long-term good, it fosters parasitic consumption, or unsustainable living. This is the source of the ecological disasters in process that now afflict our planet and threaten our future. *Susto* consumer culture drives ruthless bargains with Mother Nature, exploiting and consuming her resources, leaving her wounds for future generations to heal, devouring her in a meal-without-reciprocity that, if unchecked, leads to catastrophe. Extinction is the fate of parasites that devour their host.

Indigenous cultures understood sustainable reciprocity and made it the ceremonial basis of their lives. They saw the earth as their sustaining mother. They recognized their interdependence within the web of life. They intuited their ultimate dependence upon mysterious spiritual powers. Conscious of all the above, they lived in gratitude and humility, in the spirit of sustainable reciprocity. These understandings, which formed the ceremonial basis of indigenous culture, found high expression in shamanism.

The first initiation in my own shamanic apprenticeship was a hands-on experience of sustainable reciprocity. I had gone to the Amazon to spend three weeks working in don Antonio's large ethno-botanical gardens. I went in a spirit of humility and gratitude for being accepted as his apprentice, and for the positive impact he had already had in my life. My first task was sweeping the thick carpet of leaves from the garden floor. It took a full day. After that I would learn to wield a two-foot machete to clear the rapidly grow-ing flora from the garden's numerous medicinal herbs.

Gardening is sustainable reciprocity at its most elemental level. You give to the earth, and the earth gives back to you. I had no idea that first day as I cleared the garden paths that I was actually clear-ing my own path. I still remember how my inner state shifted as I worked that afternoon. Starting from my ordinary, busy, distracted mind, I gradually became more aware of my surroundings. I even began to see more clearly. I felt a growing spiritual and emotional connection to the life and the jungle surrounding me. I noticed that everything was profoundly alive.

I swept the fallen leaves of the towering cecropia trees that blocked the sky; the leaves and lavender flowers of the regal jacaranda tree; the fronds of the trunkless, otherworldly stilt palm; and the maroon pod-fruits of the achiote tree. As I swept, I lost all sense of time and merged with the timeless jungle. I felt nature alive and pulsing all around. And I was not separate from it. I was a crea-ture doing my part in creation, serving nature who took care of me. In those moments, sweeping leaves in the jungle seemed the most meaningful thing I had ever done. And in a way, it was.

Then, suddenly, I found myself weeping uncontrollably, sup-porting my heaving body on the broom handle, overwhelmed by a profound sense of connection with the earth, of awe at the sacred-ness of nature, of gratitude for life. The healing, life-changing expe-rience was a profound awakening to the spirit of sustainable reciprocity.

A famous Zen story tells of Master Hyakujo, who worked in the temple gardens throughout his life. When he was in his eighties, his well-meaning disciples decided that he had earned a retirement from physical labor. They also knew he would not voluntarily give up working. So one night they hid his tools. The next day, unable to find his tools, the master did not work. Nor did he eat. The day after that he again neither worked nor ate. His students got the message. That night they returned his tools. The next day he resumed his former routine. In that evening's instruction, he simply said, "No work, no food."

Master Hyakujo understood sustainable reciprocity; his work was a tangible gift, given in humility and gratitude, to life itself that gave endlessly to him. As long as he could work, he refused to violate the principle of reciprocity, to take without giving. By living the law of reciprocity, he set an example for those around him, and spirit energy flowed through him in abundance, connecting him to life, and to himself, at the highest levels. This is the example that hardworking don Antonio, so full of vitality and joy, has always set for me.

Most of us have experienced the sense of peace, balance, and calm that comes from working in a garden. This peace is the energetic fullness we access through sustainable reciprocity. All altruistic action connects us to a higher circuit of spirit energy, raising our level of consciousness and releasing us, if only briefly, from the stressful isolation of the *susto* self. When we physically serve the earth, we link up with her literal magnetic field and spirit energy, and are recharged with vitality. When we personally serve others we link up to the magnetic field, or spirit energy circuit that connects all humanity. This partly accounts for the good feeling, and the numerous health benefits, we get when we perform acts of kindness or generosity, or help someone in need.

Each of us is born an indigenous self with inherent spiritual drives or needs: to love and be loved, to act with kindness and do good to others, to contribute something of value to the world. Altruism fulfills these innate drives. As we act altruistically, we access greater energy. And we must fulfill these needs in order to be fulfilled in life. This is one of the primary conditions of being human.

This is why pets are so popular, and so good for our health. Pets allow us to experience the altruistic side of our nature without the complications that tend to characterize human relationships. The pleasurable feeling we get when we stop to pet a stray dog or cat—an act of kindness with no thought of reward—is the simple joy of expressing our deeper altruistic nature. Numerous studies and pet projects in prisons have shown that pets awaken altruistic responses and healthy self-esteem in hardened criminals, even in murderers.

Altruism is a sustainable virtue, a higher human impulse that uplifts us, others, the community, and the world. It is spirit energy in action, aligning us to *its* deepest purposes and intentions. Altruism is the best medicine for the chronic energy-depleting fears and concerns of the *susto* self. It releases deeper wellsprings of spirit energy within us. In time it leads us to fulfill our highest human potential, both as energy beings and as spiritual beings. Individuals like Mahatma Gandhi, Mother Teresa, Martin Luther King, and of course Buddha and Christ, show how higher altruism unleashes a dynamic spiritual power into the world that changes lives, and even history.

But every individual act of altruism positively impacts the world because we truly are all connected in a vast interdependent web of life. So remember the butterfly's wings, and consider what energies your own random acts of kindness might release in the world, and in you. Remember that there is infinite spirit energy, or love, in the universe, and you can have all you are willing to give away. Understand that only a collective shift to sustainable reciprocity will heal our troubled world. But this collective shift will only happen when enough individuals have made this shift. And when enough of us do, our troubled world will be healed, transformed and lifted to its next stage of spiritual evolution.

Altruism Exercise

For some of us it might seem unclear how we might get more energy by giving energy away through acts of reciprocity. Let's do a step-by-step exercise so you can experience the truth of this principle of altruism.

Begin with the Four-Step Shift, perhaps at your altar or meditation space, or in some other quiet place. Close your eyes and note for a moment how your heart feels right now and how your body feels around your heart. For most of us there is some tightness there, some constriction. That's the *susto* self keeping our hearts from being soft and open.

Now think of a person, place, or thing that has made a significant contribution to your life. You might be thinking about a special nature place of your youth where you built forts and climbed trees, or about people who have supported your dream of a new business that now produces a flourishing income for you and your family. Feel those living connections you have with others that are an integral part of your life.

Now get up from your quiet space and gather up an item that represents this special place or group, perhaps a picture of your youth in the wilds of that special nature place or some award or important memento found or given to you by others. Put that item in front of you or on your sacred altar. Close your eyes and recall all the details of why that place, or person, or people were or are so special in your life. Remember all the details, all the feelings, all the outcomes of those events. Get connected to the physical, emotional, and mental memories of those events, places, and people.

Now shift your attention to your heart. Notice how your heart, and the muscles around your heart, have softened in the glow of remembrance of something good and meaningful to you. Take the next moments to thank the people and places for those gifts to your life. Ask the spirit of that nature place or those community folk just what it is that you can do to give back. As you speak the words of gratitude in your heart, notice again how the heart and chest area relax even more. Gratitude leads to love, which opens the body, mind, and spirit even more. It is out of this love of the people, places, and things that have brought you such happiness that the heart will speak to you as to how you can perform an act of reciprocity. Your heart may tell you to organize a group to plant more trees in the park, to give youth more trees to climb on. Your heart may ask you to participate in a local wilderness conservancy group, to preserve a large space of wilderness for the generations to come. You may hear your heart tell you to offer a free meal to the indigent from your restaurant, or even to one needy person.

Now experience the mystery of the power of reciprocity. As you actualize what your heart has asked you to do, your kindness and generosity will open the hearts of others. In doing so, more spirited energy flows in this miraculous circuit of reciprocity. It's as simple as "what goes around, comes around." These simple acts awaken mutual vitality and passion by connecting a relational circuit between human beings. Where the energy circuit is completed through reciprocity, a light glows between two spirits and overflows into the world.

Many times a day I realize how much my own outer and inner life is built upon the labors of my fellow-men, both living and dead, and how earnestly I must exert myself in order to give in return as much as I have received.

—Albert Einstein

Section Three

The Five Common Energy Leaks

12

Anxiety: Separation from Self and Nature

A chronically anxious, exhausted, burnt-out caregiver" was how Rosie, an OB-GYN nurse and mother of two, described herself to me. She had come with me to the Amazon jungle in search of a deeply healing, life-changing experience. Each day at work, Rosie helped women through their intensive birthing labor. At home she tried to help her son, diagnosed with attention deficit hyperactivity disorder, manage his energy outbursts. He took Ritalin for his ADHD. She took Xanax for her anxiety.

Rosie's chronic internal feeling was "wound-up and exhausted at the same time." Her daily anxiety depleted her energy resources so completely that she would often collapse by 7 P.M., unable to enjoy the evening with her family. Anxiety also interfered with her sleep. Unable to get sufficient rest, she was frazzled every morning before she started work. Desperate to find a solution that her life had not delivered and her pharmaceuticals had not provided, she had come to the Amazon to get away from it all, hoping to "kick" Xanax, recoup her energy, and find another way to live.

We arrived in Iquitos, checked into the hotel, and then headed for a medicinal plant garden just outside the city. We would spend the first day there, before leaving for the depths of the jungle, getting acclimatized to the jungle heat. Before we even began touring the garden, Rosie announced, her face torn with weariness, anxiety, and conflict, that she was considering returning home. She felt as if she were abandoning her patients and her son.

We sat down together and I asked her what was wrong. Her anxiety spilled out as she told me how frantic her life had been prior to her departure. She now felt that this trip was a mistake; she was being irresponsible, she was really needed at home, she was abandoning her patients and her son, she said. She also confessed feeling deep apprehensions about the intensity of the jungle. She felt trapped, dreading her return to the pressures and chaos of her life at home, fearful of moving forward into the jungle experience, and under overwhelming pressure in the moment. It was pure anxiety. Trapped in her mind, dissociated from her body, she was anxiously contemplating imaginary scenarios that made her present a living hell.

I listened calmly and allowed her to express everything that was in her. Then I told her that she could trust life, herself, the choice she had made to come, the fact that she was now here, and whatever changes this trip would open up for her. I told her to relax for a few moments, take a few deep breaths, and tune in to her body. She did so. Then I told her to look around her, to see, feel, and smell the life in the jungle garden surrounding her. She was now much calmer and more present.

Then I made a suggestion: Rather than let her anxiety determine her choice, why not trust what was happening and take this journey one step at a time? She could go home at any point. But why not take a few more steps first and see what she discovered? Rosie decided stay through the medicinal garden tour and see how she felt afterward. She would consider her next step at the end of the day, back at the hotel. I knew the plants and the vibrant life force of the jungle would begin to heal her.

That afternoon Rosie's chronic stress, anxiety, and exhaustion began to shift. She opened up to feel and trust her experience in the potent jungle environment, and entered the gateway of Mother Nature, whose power heals mind, body, and spirit. As Rosie meandered through the jungle garden getting to know each plant by sight, name, and medicinal purpose and more intimately by smell and touch, her whole being began to relax. The medicine that is nature, fully alive in the Garden of Eden that is the Amazon jungle, was working in her. By the end of the day, filled to the brim with the energy and aroma of the plants and the highly oxygenated rain-forest air, Rosie had visibly changed. She decided to stay for the whole journey.

Millions of Americans, like Rosie, suffer from chronic anxiety, the most common psychological disorder in America. The best estimate is that roughly 65 percent of adults (almost 25 percent of the population) experience recurring symptoms of anxiety, which include chronic stress, fear, obsessive worry, poor concentration, irritability, anguish, dread, frequent or chronic tiredness, fatigue, sleep disorders, and physical tension. We all experience occasional symptoms of anxiety, but when any of these symptoms become chronic, *susto* is taking over.

No matter how modern and civilized we may appear, we are still natural beings forged in the wilds of nature over millions of years. Our bodies and our spirits still crave and respond to the healing powers of plants, the oxygen they produce, and the very soil out of which they grow. When we are separated from nature, we are separated from the nourishing spiritual manna of our primordial, bio-spiritual roots. Anxiety is one common side effect of this separation, though it is clearly compounded by the multifaceted stresses of modern life. Yet when we return to Mother Nature's bosom, we are replenished by her vital manna, which can heal us of much modern neurosis and even physical ailments.

The disconnection from nature and the corresponding anxiety that characterize modern life are reflected in the types and amounts of anxiety medication we take, and by the very fact that we primarily treat anxiety with chemicals. Imagine taking a child away from its mother. Then, when the child developed the natural symptoms of separation anxiety, imagine that, instead of returning it to its mother, you stunned it into apparent calmness with anxiety medications. This is how shamans like don Antonio view a pharmaceutical approach to *susto*-based ailments.

Fear is the brain's normal response to threat. Anxiety is fear that won't stop when threat has been removed or is not immediately present. By contemplating a *possible* tax audit months away; by replaying in our minds an accident we *almost* had, or did have on the freeway; by repeatedly recalling painful things someone said or did to us in the past, we trigger anxiety in the present, *now*, and *now*, and *now*. When this becomes a habit, anxiety *(susto)* has taken over our life.

Chronic anxiety is a result of an activity we are compulsively performing, either consciously or subconsciously. Chronic anxiety is a result of our meditating on, or mentally reliving, moments of pain, embarrassment, dread, or threat that occurred in the past; or rehearsing imaginary future moments that haven't happened yet, and may never happen. The blessing and the curse of humanness, of being thinking creatures, is that we *can* imagine the future and remember the past. And the future we imagine or the past we recall and relive can mean the difference between heaven and hell in the present.

A visionary, writer, poet, or artist intentionally imagines as a conscious, creative act and is uplifted in the process. Anxiety sufferers are trapped in their unconscious or compulsive negative imaginings and are tormented by the process. The torment of anxiety sufferers is not knowing how to turn off their terrible imaginings.

Part of the problem is that our reptilian rear-brains are still doing in this high-tech modern age what they were designed to do in the primordial jungles and savannahs of our evolutionary forebears—trigger hardwired fight-or-flight responses to alert us to potential danger in a world of predators, brutal nature, and tribal wars. Our hair-trigger, fear-based proto-human brain is alive and well and functioning out of context in the twenty-first century. And the stress is making many of us ill. The world has changed, but our conditioned responses remain as primitive as our limbic brains. Today's complex, unprecedented stresses can evoke counterproductive, even self-destructive neurological responses from this primitive brain that still drives us. The irrational limbic brain interprets unmanageable complexity as a threat.

"Freezing" is a classic neurological response to perceived threat, especially when one feels helpless in the face of a threat or challenge. Some people literally cripple themselves psychologically to avoid perceived threats that may not even be real. To the limbic brain, all anxiety has survival value. But anxiety disconnects us from life, and leaves us isolated and in fear.

Many triggers for anxiety are unconscious, or semiconscious. When a limbic anxiety trigger is switched, our neurochemistry turns on our stress hormones. Then the "higher" newer brain area, the neocortex, evaluates the situation, seeking reasons to explain the stress announced by the irrational limbic brain. When you are anxious, you "explain" your anxiety to yourself in a seemingly plausible way that is often quite irrational. This is what Rosie was doing as she told me why she wanted to leave the jungle to which she had come seeking healing, and return home *to the very life that was the source of her chronic anxiety.*

You can always find reasons to be worried, and those with chronic anxiety usually do. But as the logic of Rosie's rationale shows, anxiety uses logic in a completely irrational fashion. And its "solutions" usually increase stress, rather than solve or relieve it.

Part of the problem is that, as current neurobiology shows, we unconsciously adapt to, and even become addicted to, unhealthy (and healthy) states of mind and emotion. Chronic anxiety, chronic depression, and other negative emotional states may be unconsciously sought out because they are familiar and we are used to them. And we may perversely crave the familiar, even when it makes us miserable, and habitually or compulsively seek it out or restimulate it.

Emotional and psychological healing requires that new, healthy patterns of thinking and feeling be cultivated in place of old, unhealthy ones. Fortunately, timeless nature, which includes our own psyche and spirit, is ever ready to provide a cure.

Shaman don Antonio joined Rosie and me the next day and we boarded the boat that would take us deep into the Amazon's emerald forests. Don Antonio sat in the front of the boat with his back to the bow, facing us. Now, on the boat heading down the river, Rosie's anxiety returned. For a few moments don Antonio looked deeply into her eyes, which were full of fear.

"She has *susto*," he said softly.

Don Antonio was looking with a shaman's eyes, seeing in her the ravages of years of stress hormones in her body, mind, and spirit. Now he asked Rosie to tell him more about her life and the emotions pent-up in her heart. He listened patiently, nodding and occasionally responding as she unleashed a torrent of pent-up fears, heartaches, and concerns that the Xanax had numbed, perhaps, but left unhealed. Finally she stopped, seeming visibly relieved. Then don Antonio asked her if she would stop taking Xanax while she was in the jungle. He knew the power of the jungle's medicine and did not want it to be diminished by her Western pharmaceuticals. Rosie agreed.

"Anxiety and fear are forms of *susto*," don Antonio explained to Rosie. "*Susto* causes spirit loss—a part of you disappears. It is possible to be frightened to death over time. When *susto* is not healed, it may allow fear to become our continuous state. We lose faith in the goodness of life. We become anxious about getting up in the morning, about going to our work, about our encounters and relationships with others, even about being alive. This is not normal. But it may come to seem normal. And when what is abnormal becomes normal, when anxiety becomes our daily companion and drugs become our daily solution, we grow weak, hopeless, and disconnected from life. We lose our vitality and passion. We are robbed of our spirit. We no longer breathe in the force of life. Notice how you are breathing now, in little puffs that barely keep you alive. I see this new form of *susto* in many of the Westerners I meet these days.

"But don't worry," he added. "You are now surrounded by the best medicine there is—the jungle. Her fresh food, water, and air will nourish your body. Her aroma, her sounds and colors, will soothe your mind and restore your spirit. Her spirit energy will fill you with new life."

Rosie and I listened attentively, feeling the palpable peace of nature and her spirit energy enfolding us. Over the next week, through simple activities and moments, Rosie was transformed before my eyes. Every morning at dawn the three of us took a dip in the waters of an Amazon River tributary in front of our bungalow. Don Antonio said the power of living waters was highly energizing, and that the electric eels and giant anacondas that lived in these waters give it a special charge. He also had Rosie breathe fully and deeply several times a day to absorb the vital spirit energy in the oxygen.

Each morning, after a delicious breakfast of juicy papaya and fresh catfish, we'd lounge for an hour in the hammock before the heat of the day. Then we'd go for a silent meditative walk with don Antonio along the shaded trails under a rooftop canopy of trees that blotted out the sky, absorbing with all of our senses the jungle's vital force. A light, refreshing lunch consisting of chicken, fresh pineapple juice, and crisp cucumbers was generally followed by a long siesta, prompted both by the meal and the jungle heat.

After our siesta, we'd often work for a few hours in don Antonio's jungle garden. Then we'd go walking the trails again, gathering various aromatic herbs and flowers for our *limpia*, a healing herbal bath. After we immersed our sticky bodies in the river, don Antonio administered the *limpia*, pouring over our heads a large bowl of water soaked in the aromatic flowers and herbs. This cleansing ritual removed all negative energies gathered during the day and infused our bodies, minds, and spirits with the life-giving energies of these healing herbs.

Then the three of us would sit on the porch of our jungle house, looking out over the river, sipping on refreshing lemony *hierba luisa*, which we know as lemongrass tea. Afterward, soothed and energized by the *limpia*, the tea, and the vibrant jungle itself, we ate our last meal of the day, usually fish soup, a local favorite.

Sunset signaled time for bed, as sunrise signaled time to rise and shine. There is nothing like the Amazon jungle night, being lulled to deep, refreshing sleep by the sounds of mating frogs, diverse insect noises, and the strange and enchanting cries of nocturnal birds.

Over the days of our retreat, all the components of the Four-Step Shift were applied in one form or another, in most of the gateways. Rosie paid attention to her body and its feelings and emotion; she exercised daily, conducting her physical energy through hiking, swimming, and gardening, while continuing to relax, feel, and breathe deeply and often. She paid attention to her thoughts and the feelings they produced, noticing and releasing anxious *susto* thoughts and letting her deepening connection to her indigenous self and the pleasure of nature surrounding her naturally calm her mind. She remembered, and was reminded often, that she was part of a web of life; that like the rest of nature, she was in fact being lived and breathed by the Source of all life. By relaxing in this awareness many times in the day and by performing all of her activities as ways of receiving and conducting spirit energy in interdependence with nature, Rosie's life naturally fell into balance with nature and with Spirit. And this reestablished and deepened her connection with her indigenous self, and with Spirit, producing a deep and lasting shift in her awareness and her perspective on her life. One result was a healing that her pharmaceutical medications had failed to deliver.

These things occur naturally if we spend enough time in nature. The living power and spirit of nature parts the veils from our eyes and reveals our own nature to us. And this is inherently healing.

"Trust Spirit and trust nature," don Antonio had said early in the week. "They both live within you. And don't forget the plants."

Don Antonio was right. In only a week, Rosie's healing was apparent. Nature was restoring her health and vitality. Her face was now relaxed and rested. Her eyes were clear and open. There was a new light and energy in her. She was off the Xanax, and into life. I loved the sound of her lively laughter and her cheerful "Good night!" after she crawled into our mosquito netting, ready for another restful night's sleep.

The last night of our stay in the jungle, Rosie dreamed that out of her Xanax bottle sprouted fragrant flowers, succulent fruits, and nurturing greens, all surrounded by a warm, golden glow. The power of this vision stayed with her all night, filling her body and her heart with ecstasy and peace. In the morning Rosie shared her dream with don Antonio. He was very pleased.

"The medicine of the jungle has planted itself inside you." He smiled. "Remember to preserve these feelings of peace, connection, and love of life that you have found here in the jungle. Nurture this peace like a delicate flower. Make it your *disciplina*. Water it with silence, with the sounds and smells and life force of nature. Remember that this peace of nature *is* your nature. When you return home, find this same *energia espirita* in nature where you live. Take a few minutes each day to find it and feel it where it lives inside of you. And drink often from this Source of life."

Rosie fidgeted for a moment, already imagining her return to her stress-filled life.

"Don Antonio," she said, "I'm afraid when I go back I'll fall into my old life again, back into my Xanax bottle."

With gentle humor, don Antonio put a sprig of aromatic wild basil under her nose.

"Whenever you feel anxious," he said, "don't turn on the TV. Don't think about your problems. Feel the breath of life that is always coming in and going out of you. Take an herbal bath or sit quietly and sip a relaxing tea. Get up and go outside. Smell a lovely flower, walk in the woods, lie on the grass and look at the sky. The Earth has an energy field that heals and recharges you. Even to stand barefoot on a patch of grass, or lean against a tree, changes your state. Stop every day and feel the presence of nature with all of your senses. And remember that you are part of her. Let this awareness penetrate you, all the way into your bones. It will always restore you. Look how nature has healed you here in only one week because you took time to stop and drink her *energia espirita*. Make this your prescription instead of pills that do not heal, but only numb your pain.

"Nature is a garden blooming from the ocean of spirit. You are a flower in the garden of nature. Find ways to keep your roots in her so that her life force flows through you. This will cure your *susto*. It will give you boundless energy and a passion for life. It will flow through you into your son, your family, and your patients. You will become a healing force to those around you. We are not meant to live separated from nature, spreading the *susto* that then consumes us. We are meant to live feeling nature's spirit as our own spirit, our very self, and letting that flow through us."

Rosie returned to her hectic personal and professional life back home. As she told me later, "Everything has changed, and nothing has changed. I'm still me, but I feel like a different person." Something had shifted in her consciousness, and in her relationship to her life. No longer a deer in the headlights reduced to chemical remedies, she was ready to take on her life and her own healing with proactive measures. From this new disposition, she found it remarkably easy to continue doing the things that had healed her during her jungle adventure—eat more fresh foods, relax and breathe more deeply, take regular brisk walks in nature, communing with its silence and its life-giving oxygen. She even planted a garden in memory of her rain-forest experience and what the shaman had taught her. She says, "Gardening for me is now more effective than Xanax. I'm at peace when I'm there. It helps me cope with the day."

Rosie remains Xanax-free to date. Her son is being tapered off the Ritalin as I write, under her watch-care, using don Antonio's "nature cure." As don Antonio suggested, peace, like *susto,* is also transmitted from person to person.

Fortunately, we don't all need to go to the Amazon jungle to find our healing. Chapter Seventeen, "Nature's Energy Medicine Chest," will help you design a healing program for anxiety, or any other condition, incorporating all of the gateways and the Four-Step Shift.

13

Depression: A Loss of Soul,
a Rebirth of Self

Depression afflicts an estimated 20 million Americans each year, and it affects the lives of many millions more—of family members, friends, and co-workers. Depression, the most frequently diagnosed psychiatric illness, the leading cause of suicide, and a major factor in numerous other ailments, touches most of us at some point in our lives.

Because it is frequently associated with and disguised by other symptoms and conditions, it often goes unrecognized and undiagnosed. Depression's secondary symptoms may include loss of appetite, loss of weight, even anorexia; compulsive eating, weight gain and obesity; lethargy, apathy, low energy, and chronic fatigue; insomnia and/or excessive sleeping; feelings of shame, guilt, inadequacy, and low self-esteem; loss of mental clarity, diminished concentration, and even Alzheimer's disease; loss of motivation and incapacitation of the will; chronic pessimism, negativity, and irritability; loss of interest in things that once brought enjoyment; a heaviness or flattening of the personality; substance abuse (includes food, alcohol, drugs, and TV); psychosomatic ailments such as headaches, stomach and intestinal ailments, hypochondria; and more. Many of the above symptoms are also unconscious behaviors through which the depressed person is attempting to cope with, avoid, or deaden painful feelings.

Depression is not grief, sadness, or discouragement. These are natural and common responses to traumatic, painful, or disappointing events. But when these feelings persist, deepen, and become chronic, when grief becomes despair and discouragement becomes hopelessness, and when these moods begin to define our personality, color our view of life, and diminish our vitality, then we are clinically depressed.

Not surprisingly, antidepressants are the most frequently prescribed, and the most overprescribed, drugs in America. Zoloft, for example, ranked number five in the number of prescriptions dispensed in 2003, earning $2,878,686,000 in revenue from 32,718,000 prescriptions.

It's an accepted fact that antidepressants don't heal depression. They help patients manage or alleviate the symptoms of depression, but they do not address or heal the emotional, psychological, and spiritual roots of depression, or resolve the more practical issues and factors that may be causing or contributing to the depression. And, increasingly, the FDA is coming out with stern warnings on the dangers of antidepressants, especially to children and teenagers. The opening line of an Associated Press news release from October 20, 2004, reads:

"All antidepressants must carry a 'black box' warning, the government's strongest safety alert, linking the drugs to increased suicidal thoughts and behavior among children and teens taking them, the Food and Drug Administration said Friday."

We can be fairly certain that aspirin will relieve a headache, sore muscles, aches and pains. But a recent Rand Corporation research study involving 1,200 clinically depressed patients in 46 hospitals around the United States over a period of 18 months found no improvement in nearly half of those treated with a combination of therapy and antidepressants. Clearly, the efficacy of these drugs, and our current treatment models for depression, are inadequate.

What Causes Depression?

Humpty Dumpty sat on a wall
Humpty Dumpty had a great fall
All the king's horses and all the king's men
Couldn't put Humpty together again.

Science links depression to an imbalance in our brain's biochemistry, with a reduction in neurotransmitters like serotonin and norepinephrine, and with a malfunctioning of the neural circuits that regulate our moods, sleep, appetite, sex drive, willpower, and cognitive functions. It also tells us that depression can be passed on genetically as an inherited biological disposition, meaning that we may carry a probability for depression in our genes.

But biochemical imbalances in the brain and genetic predisposition are not the only causes of depression. If they were, mere pharmaceutical readjustment of our brain chemistry would cure depression. But it doesn't. At best, antidepressants suppress or diminish overwhelming feelings of despair and "clear the fog," allowing the severely depressed person to function again.

Psychology tells us the following about depression: A depressed parent may predispose a child, emotionally and psychologically, to depression later in life. Depression in adults may be triggered by any one event or a combination of painful events or prolonged stressful situations such as job loss, divorce, a death of a loved one, a major illness or injury, emotional abuse, joblessness, poverty, loneliness, and more. Poor social and relationship skills and an inability

WHY ANTIDEPRESSANTS MAY NOT WORK

The cutting edge of antidepressant prescription therapy is in the category of drugs termed the SSRIs (selective serotonin reuptake inhibitors) like the top sellers Prozac, Paxil, and Zoloft. The theory behind their invention was called "the amine hypothesis." This hypothesis states that depression may be caused by low levels of certain brain chemicals (neurotransmitters) called amines (serotonin, as an example). The proposed mechanism of action of the SSRIs is to raise the level of serotonin, thereby relieving depression. In fact, it's only hypothetical that serotonin levels are low in the brains of depressed people. SSRIs don't always work, and they can have serious side effects for some. Overall, they represent a "false energy" in that for most patients, the depression returns when medication is stopped.

to relax and manage or release stress may also contribute to depression. Everyone has a tipping point where the stresses and shocks of life exceed the capacity to endure them. Given sufficient or prolonged pressure, or the wrong combination of stressful circumstances, anyone may fall into depression.

Modern existential psychologists tell us the depressed person's crippling sense of hopelessness, futility, or despair reflects a loss of meaning in life, which reflects a corresponding loss of meaning in modern secular culture and society. Most of us live by meanings inherited from our culture and family—ideas, roles, and purposes like being a good citizen, a good parent, a good spouse, a good provider, a good soldier, a good teacher, a successful businessman, and the like. In depression, these conventional roles and meanings become empty. They no longer provide the motivation or the energy to go on as before. The depressed person is unable to live with conviction, to participate energetically in life. The severely depressed person may be unable to get out of bed. Energetically depleted and spiritually broken, life is no longer a sustainable proposition for the depressed person.

It is ultimately mysterious why one person falls into depression while another in similar circumstances does not. We all inherit a variety of genetic traits and tendencies from our parents. We are all significantly shaped or "predispositioned" by their behavior and emotional patterns, and by our childhood trials and traumas. We are all impacted by present life stresses. All of these and more continually affect our brain's biochemistry. But not all of us are tipped into crippling depression, robbed of a sense of life's meaning and our own value as human beings.

What is important is to know that it is possible for a depressed person to tap the inner wellsprings of spirit, access the spirit energy that is the source of true healing, and be restored to new life.

Shamans have much to say on this matter.

A Shamanic View of Depression

Shamans view depression as a spiritual condition with two aspects:

First: Depression is perceived as a loss of soul, a leak or wound in our spirit through which our life force has drained away. It is the collapse of a *susto* self that has reached its limits and can no longer bear up under the pressures and stresses of life. The depressed person has withdrawn into a cocoon of shock, despair, or numbness the way a sick or wounded animal crawls off into the bushes to heal or die. In this view, the depression is a natural, instinctive response to unbearable stress, pain, loss, and helplessness. Some shamans say the soul of a severely depressed person has literally left the body. Indeed, depression's numbing of emotion, paralysis of will, and inability to face and embrace life are a kind of soullessness, or living death.

Second: Depression is seen as the soul's necessary, perhaps unavoidable, withdrawal from "normal" participation in the outer world, a journey inward *for the purposes of healing, renewal, and transformation*. In this view, depression is a kind of self-protective cocoon from which a new self will hopefully emerge. This positive view points both to the healing of depression (or any other severe psychological affliction) and to the birth of a new self and a new life. It is a winter of the soul that leads to spring.

The idea of spiritual death leading to a rebirth of self is found in the myths and religions of almost every culture, from the phoenix rising from the ashes to the death and resurrection of Christ. And a cognitive reframing of depression from a Western "pathology only" view to the shamanic death-and-rebirth view is inherently healing.

Unlike Western medicine, shamanism recognizes that difficult and painful inward journeys, including so-called pathological emotional and psychological disorders, may be essential parts of a process leading to spiritual transformation and rebirth. A shaman trusts the soul's reasons for withdrawing into non-ordinary states of consciousness. He helps the "patient" understand the spiritual nature of his illness. And he guides him to connect, in practical and spiritual ways, to those inner spiritual resources that facilitate healing, renewal, and the emergence of a new, sustainable self. This approach allows us to relate to our own non-ordinary states and processes in a healthier way that produces healthier outcomes.

In my shamanic memoir, *Jungle Medicine*, I tell the story of my experiences with the shaman don Antonio. When I first became his apprentice I was recovering from cancer, divorce, and in the midst of a profound emotional and spiritual crisis that included a major depression. Western medicine had utterly failed in restoring my spirit. But don Antonio led me through my ordeal by helping me to shift my consciousness from *susto* to experience the native peace of my indigenous self. This involved a shift in perspective on my crisis from a fearful vision of catastrophe and doom to an expanded shamanic vision of death and rebirth. He also helped me to establish healthy disciplines in the gateways that connected me to the spirit energy that heals. With his help, I emerged from my ordeal stronger, wiser, and more connected to Spirit than I had ever been before. It was indeed the birth of a new self, and a new life.

Depression and other emotional and psychological afflictions can be life shattering. But shamans believe the soul sometimes chooses pain and shattering disillusionment in order to grow into greater wholeness. An old life is sloughed off like a snake shedding its skin, and a new and greater life is revealed. But the soul must choose this in the midst of the ordeal. And it can do this only when the armor of our old *susto* personality has been penetrated. Our human personality is not our true nature. Spirit is our true nature. And sometimes the old needs to die so that the new can be reborn.

What Is the Cure?

If depression is the collapse of an unsustainable *susto* self, then the "cure" for depression is the birth of a new, sustainable self. This birth involves progressive, and sometimes sudden, shifts in consciousness that deepen our connection to the Source of spirit energy within, and that initiate healing and transformation.

The modern psychotherapeutic model for healing depression involves progressive and often painstaking inner and outer work with the help of a psychotherapist. In this model, exploring and addressing the emotional and psychological roots of depression while making progressive behavioral changes facilitates healing. For the severely depressed, antidepressants can be a useful phase in this process, giving us temporary relief from unbearable pain and allowing us to get our feet back on the ground and begin moving forward.

The shamanic model and the psychotherapeutic model for depression and healing have similarities and key differences. To a shaman, depression is the *susto* self at the end of its rope. It has run out of energy and the will to go on. All its inner resources are exhausted and it cannot heal itself. It has no solutions, and never did. The paralysis of depression is unconditional surrender to fear. The *susto* self is always choosing fear, and so is incapable of truly choosing life.

But hidden within this shattered, separated *susto* self the shaman sees an indigenous self, already whole and one with Spirit. To a shaman, the healing of depression is not the healing of the *susto* self, nor is it a painstaking rebuilding of a shattered self through inner and outer work. It is a progressive rebirth or awakening of this true, sustainable self. Inner and outer work are still essential for healing, but they are not seen as the Source of healing.

To accomplish this healing, the shaman invokes a primary power which the psychotherapist does not—the power of Spirit. And he calls on the spirit of the patient to choose life. He knows that Spirit heals our depression when we make a decisive choice for life. He knows that when our spirit calls on Spirit, it comes. It enters into us and begins to do the work of healing and renewal that we cannot do for ourselves. Spirit is always waiting and willing to do this work in us, but our *susto* self is not open to Spirit. It is always turning away, pursuing other things and goals in life.

This knowledge is the basis of shamanism, which is a path of calling Spirit into the material world for the purposes of healing, creation, and transformation.

Depression and Spiritual Healing

Ellen, a thirty-seven-year-old corporate manager, had been struggling with cycles of depression since her mid-teens. She had done much inner work over the years, reading numerous self-help books, exhaustively "analyzing and processing" her difficult childhood, doing journal work, seeing a therapist, attending motivational and transformational seminars. She maintained healthy disciplines in key gateways, eating a healthy diet, getting regular exercise, drinking eight to twelve glasses of water daily. All these things helped her to stay motivated and generally upbeat—except when her depressions came, which they did periodically. She even got a prescription for Prozac, which she took on occasions when her depression seemed overwhelming.

Then a good friend recommended that she see a visiting shaman who had a gift for connecting people to Spirit. Ellen went to see the shaman about her depression. In their meeting, which took less than an hour, he explained to her that Spirit had power to heal her, literally to lift her out of her depression into a new place in her life. But to be fully healed, he said, she must begin living her life on a new basis, in relationship with Spirit, by whatever name she called it. He said she must trust Spirit with her life, and draw on its power daily through inner disciplines of prayer and meditation. He asked her if she wanted this healing and this new relationship with Spirit. She said yes. And she meant it.

He then performed a brief ritual in which he prayed over her and called on Spirit to come into her and heal her depression. Ellen silently prayed this for herself and opened to receive Spirit, which she called God. Ellen felt something shift in her. She sensed a spiritual presence and felt hopeful for her healing.

After the session she went home. Her depression lifted over the course of the afternoon. In the coming days it didn't return. She began doing daily prayer and meditation, inviting Spirit/God to keep coming in. Her sense of a spiritual presence in her life deepened. She knew something remarkable was happening. Weeks passed and her depression didn't return. Then one afternoon she felt the familiar gloomy feeling that always preceded her depression.

"I became aware that I could slip back into my depression if I let myself," she says. "But knew I didn't have to. I didn't want to. I saw that I had a choice. I said no to the depression. Then I did a prayer and asked Spirit to come in. And it did."

Ellen calls this her moment of choice. That was several years ago. She's had many moments of choice since then. But she chooses Spirit now. She now lives on the basis of this relationship. And her depression hasn't returned.

"I look the same," she says. "But I'm a different person in many ways. I live on the basis of very different principles. I have no interest in going back to my old life."

Ellen continues to access spirit energy through healthy disciplines in the gateways. But her main discipline is choosing and relying on Spirit as the foundation of her life. And she increasingly conducts its power through prayer, meditation, and service to others. She says these disciplines are more beneficial, healing, and energizing than any antidepressant. And she's happier, and healthier, than she's ever been.

If you suffer from depression, you can begin taking simple actions in the gateways that will shift your consciousness and infuse your body and mind with spirit energy. Things like exercise and proper breathing and hydration will make a difference in the way you feel. And they are an important part of your healing process.

But your authentic choice for Spirit is the most powerful action you can take. You don't have to wait for a shaman to come to town. Not only shamans work with Spirit to help others. Spirit is universal. It works through many people of many paths and faiths. It works with everyone who chooses it. And if you choose, it will work directly with you.

The best way to begin the process of healing depression is to do the Four-Step Shift into your indigenous self. Then find a place in you, in your spirit, that wants to be healed, that wants to live a new life on a new foundation; that wants to know and be transformed by Spirit.

You will also need to begin taking simple healing actions in the gateways. These actions include basic exercise, complete breathing, drinking sufficient water, eating a healthy diet, and doing conscious relaxation, prayer, meditation, or spiritual inquiry. Each action you perform is a choice for life. Each action is medicine.

The guidelines in Chapter Seventeen, "Nature's Energy Medicine Chest," will help you to design a simple program and support structure that works for you, that fits into your schedule and meets your needs. We also recommend that you reread Laura's story in Chapter Seven, "The Food Gateway," and apply the somatic awareness process presented there to deal with the feelings of depression you may be struggling with. But most important, continue to call on Spirit daily to come in and do its work of healing in you. And it will.

We end this chapter with a summary checklist to help you in your process of healing and rebirth:

• Trust that depression, or any other emotional or psychological illness, is a spiritual process, a winter of the self that can lead to spring.

• Trust that a new self is being born in you through this process.

• Trust the process of life itself, in you and around you.

• Trust the power of Spirit that is the Source of all healing and all life.

• To heal depression, each day find the place in yourself that is willing to choose life. Do this in prayer or meditation. Remember, your choice for life, and your commitment to your own healing, are decisive factors in overcoming depression.

• Begin taking simple healing actions in the gateways. You draw spirit energy in through simple daily disciplines such as walking, complete breathing, relaxing, being in nature, and meditation or prayer.

• Identify any unmet needs, unhealed wounds, and underlying issues and stresses that may be related to your depression. Begin taking simple, progressive steps to address these things. But do not make your healing dependent on their resolution. Your healing can begin, and even be accomplished, before, or whether or not, these issues are resolved.

• Begin a process of self-examination. Note areas of personal weakness, negative or self-defeating patterns of thinking and behavior that may have made you vulnerable to depression. Begin to improve and develop in those areas. But don't beat yourself up or engage in unhealthy self-criticism.

• As often as you can, engage in responsible work, in meaningful human relationships, and in altruistic action.

• If your struggle with depression is more than you can manage alone, find a good therapist who will support your soul and spirit as well as address your mind and your life issues. Or find a wise friend or mentor whom you trust and can talk with openly.

• At least once a week, be spontaneous. Do something on the spur of the moment that brings you into contact with others or with new experiences. It may be something as simple as taking a walk through your neighborhood, seeing a movie, going to your local YMCA for a swim or a sauna, or serving at a local homeless shelter. Be creative, and adventurous! Take life by surprise! See how good it feels.

• Remember that you are part of a vast, interconnected web of life. Winter passes, and dead grasses and barren trees bloom with new life each spring. You are part of that life, and you can access its rejuvenating power. Choose life with your spirit, and your spring will come.

14

Insomnia: Mastering Sleep and the Four-Step Healing Shift

In the Amazon, when children cannot sleep at night, shamans say the spirit of fear is keeping them awake. Shamans treat this form of *susto*, which we call insomnia, with a prayer, a relaxing bath, a soothing song, a gentle touch. In the West, millions of insomniacs take sleeping pills that do not cure their condition. Many become dependent or addicted, while never learning the most basic relaxation skills that would make all the difference.

An estimated 30 to 50 percent of adult Americans experience occasional, recurring, or chronic insomnia, which includes: having trouble falling asleep, waking in the night (in some cases repeatedly) and having trouble going back to sleep, waking too early in the morning and being unable to return to sleep, waking from apparently normal sleep feeling tired, and other variations. Common daytime effects of insomnia include low energy; fatigue; difficulty concentrating and paying attention; impaired memory, learning, and comprehension; diminished motor skills; anxiety; irritability; feeling socially off balance; having difficulty being present with others. Studies show that insomniacs have a higher rate of car accidents and diminished work productivity. But it's not only insomniacs who suffer impaired functioning and health. Sleep deprivation is epidemic in our culture.

As we write this chapter there is a story in the news about a pilot for a major world airline falling asleep for half an hour in flight in the presence of an inspector. A quick search on the Web brought up numerous other articles discussing the widespread problem of fatigued pilots napping during flights. This would come as no surprise to sleep researchers, who know that travelers and shift workers have higher rates of insomnia than the average population. Senior citizens, menopausal women, and adolescent, teenage, and college-level students also suffer high rates of insomnia and sleep deprivation.

A National Sleep Foundation survey found that only 15 percent of teens are getting the recommended 8.5 hours of sleep needed for optimum functioning. College students often average less sleep than teenagers. The consequences of youth sleep deprivation include emotional difficulties, impaired attention and poor academic performance, and other effects that contribute to much worse problems. Recent studies show that chronic insomnia or habitual lack of sleep can produce symptoms of attention deficit disorder and contribute to a variety of ailments such as depression, anxiety, and even obesity, for which medications are prescribed that may aggravate the root problems of which the above symptoms are by-products. Mary Carskadon of Brown University, who studies the sleeping habits of children, finds that children who don't get sufficient sleep are often below-average students, are less likely to do well at sports, and are more likely to have emotional problems than their peers who do get enough sleep. And a recent study of automobile accidents found that nearly half of those who fell asleep while driving were under twenty-five years old.

Drugs Don't Cure Insomnia

Medical conditions such as arthritis, kidney and cardiopulmonary diseases, asthma, hyperthyroidism, chronic pain, sleep apnea, Parkinson's disease, and more do contribute to insomnia. Such medical conditions may require pharmaceutical treatment, but not exclusively. And if you have insomnia, a sleeping pill is not a wise first option.

In his exceptional book *Say Good Night to Insomnia*, Harvard researcher Greg D. Jacobs, Ph.D., tells us that "sleeping pills lose their effectiveness after six weeks of regular use." He writes that "over-the-counter sleep aids are no more effective than a sugar pill." And yet, he notes, many insomnia sufferers take sleeping pills for months and more, or use over-the-counter sleep aids, and fall asleep. Why is this? "Because the placebo effect is at work!" he says. *Placebo* is a word that points to the mind's mysterious capacity to heal. Yet there are better ways to access the healing powers of the mind than taking ineffective or disruptive medications.

Numerous studies show that sleeping pills (and other drugs) aggravate and perpetuate insomnia rather than cure it. Chemical "sleep aids" prevent deep, natural, rejuvenating sleep. They set up and promote chemical, emotional, and psychological dependency patterns. They do not heal the stress and the inability to relax and release stress that lie at the root of most insomnia. Research also indicates that imbalances in other gateways—poor dietary habits, lack of exercise, relationship problems, job stress, insufficient oxygenation and hydration—may cause or contribute to insomnia.

Unaware of, or unfamiliar with, effective alternative, nonchemical solutions to many ailments, most physicians automatically prescribe standard medications that are merely "symptom suppressive" and that frequently trigger negative side effects. (If you are currently on sleeping medication or medication for anxiety or depression, you can still benefit from the deep relaxation/somatic awareness method presented in this chapter. A recent review of 123 controlled medication studies and 33 behavioral interventions for insomnia concluded that while medications can be effective in the short term, behavioral changes produced more sustained results. And you might consider a progressive elimination program for your current medication in conjunction with this method, in consultation with an open-minded physician.)

Why Sleep Is Important

All studies confirm that sufficient sleep is crucial for optimum physical, emotional, and psychological well-being. In deep sleep our body and mind come to rest; we release emotional stress; blood flows to our entire musculature, cleansing, oxygenating, replenishing, and energizing the body; and our immune system kicks into high gear, fighting infection and illness and healing injuries.

During REM sleep, our brain nightly processes, memorizes, and digests information absorbed during the day. Not surprisingly, in infancy, when our learning and growth curves are the steepest, we average 14.5 hours sleep per 24, with more REM sleep than at any other period of life. In the first months and years of infancy, we are processing and digesting an overwhelming amount of new impressions and information, and also undergoing extraordinary physical growth and transformation.

From Stress to Sleeplessness: The Slippery Slope of Insomnia

Studies show that sleep is an automatically self-regulating function. When we are sleep deprived, we quickly and automatically enter

WHY SLEEPING PILLS DON'T WORK: A FALSE SENSE OF SLEEP

The benzodiazepine class of prescription sleeping pills (Restoril, Halcion, Doral, for example) are popular among physicians. However, there are some drawbacks. They can induce dependency, and may cause morning "hangovers" and grogginess. They can also dramatically alter the normal sleep pattern by reducing REM sleep, leaving you more tired in the morning. Taking benzodiazepines for more than a few days can cause "rebound insomnia," meaning that you might have trouble sleeping after you stop taking the benzodiazepines. Prescription and over-the-counter sleep medications give you less than the refreshing, rejuvenating sleep you need for optimum health and energy.

the sleep level that replenishes us the most and stay there, catching up for as long as we need. Our body and mind do this intelligently, without our awareness.

But stress, physical ailments, and the increasing complexity, tensions, and demands of modern life can interfere with our sleep cycles. Also, the quality of our sleep declines from middle age on. For a variety of reasons, growing numbers of people are experiencing diminished or impaired sleep capacity, making sleep—the most natural, effortless rejuvenating function after breathing—a stressful nightly preoccupation for millions of Americans.

We've seen in previous chapters how thoughts generate emotional and biochemical responses that affect our moods, our perceptions, our energy levels, our immune system, and our health. Thoughts can be stress producing, neutral, stress releasing, or energizing and healing. Our habitual thought patterns significantly shape our inner and outer life. And what the mind does at night when we're lying in bed before sleep it has probably been doing by day, unnoticed.

The problem of insomnia is the problem of *susto*. Insomnia is *susto* working the graveyard shift, keeping us awake, restless, anxious, or worried. When insomnia becomes chronic, our thoughts and fears are often *about* insomnia: "I can't go to sleep." "I have to go to sleep!" "My insomnia is getting worse!" "It's making me ill." "I'm going to be exhausted tomorrow."

Initial stress is often healthy feedback, an early signal for us to deal with inner or outer pressure or problems. When we habitually ignore or adapt to stress, more serious problems may develop. Insomnia may indicate important unresolved issues that we need to address. It may be a symptom of depression, anxiety, or some specific unresolved life issue. To discern underlying or contributing factors, it can be helpful to keep a journal of the kinds of thoughts and emotions that occur during the day, and also at night while you're unable to sleep. Note any stressful thoughts and concerns that regularly intrude in the day, and at night when you're trying to fall asleep. Your insomnia may be pointing you to issues you need to address or heal. So pay attention. Get the message. Do the work of healing out of bed rather than mulling over problems in bed.

Going to bed worrying about anything, including whether or not you will fall asleep, or following your restless mind wherever it goes stimulates sleeplessness. Bedtime is the time to relax consciously and release problems and tensions. Until we can do this reliably at will, our peace of mind, and our sleeping patterns, may be at the mercy of outer events or be sabotaged by unconscious stress patterns. We can't eliminate all sources of stress from our lives, but we can develop somatic awareness skills that allow us to recognize and release stress.

Sleep is an involuntary function. You can't "make" it happen. The best you can do is to allow it by not interfering, consciously or unconsciously. Studies show that trying to fall asleep delays or prevents sleep by producing the equivalent of performance anxiety. In *Say Good Night to Insomnia,* Dr. Greg Jacobs tells of a sleep study in which some subjects were told a cash prize would be given to whoever could fall asleep the fastest. These "motivated" subjects took three times longer to fall asleep than the main group. Apparently, not even money can buy sleep.

Fortunately, the dark cloud of insomnia has a silver lining that more than makes up for sleep lost. When built-up stress erupts in insomnia, it also offers an opportunity to heal the deeper roots of *susto* from which it springs. This healing requires learning the sustainable skill of deep relaxation to release stress, recharge our energy, and shift our state of consciousness.

With minimal practice, entering deep states of relaxation becomes a bona fide skill, repeatable at will. There are monks and shamans who, instead of sleeping at night, train themselves to remain awake in deep meditation or prayer. Those who master this discipline live healthy, dynamic lives in high levels of spiritual consciousness. Is their lack of sleep insomnia? Or are they awake in a different perspective?

Cognitive Reframing

The cure for insomnia begins with a shift of perspective, similar to that which these monks and shamans undergo in order to stay awake all night in altered states of consciousness. They don't turn out the lights at night hoping either to fall or not to fall asleep. They focus on a practice that produces a rejuvenating, life-transforming shift in awareness. They reframe the purpose of their night in a way that allows them to accomplish that purpose effectively.

Modern psychology calls this initial redefining shift in context "cognitive reframing." Finding a new meaning or purpose in an activity, situation, or problem changes our perspective on it, our relationship to it, and its effect on us. Cognitive reframing done in deep somatic awareness shifts our perspective and our emotional and biochemical state. Such a shift, which is the key to curing insomnia, is also the shift from *susto* to the indigenous self.

Here is our recommendation: For the next month, reframe bedtime as a time to practice the pleasurable, healing, rejuvenating skill of deep relaxation, which is mastering somatic awareness. Think of it this way: "Lucky me! I'm going to transformational night school on full scholarship!"

Mastering deep relaxation is mastering the shift into your indigenous self. It is the solution to insomnia, because insomnia is *susto*. Mastering deep relaxation yields profound benefits even if your insomnia is linked to a physiological problem like sleep apnea, an illness, an injury, or substance addiction. (Though in such cases you should consult a physician and/or a sleep-disorder center.)

The relaxation method in this chapter will enable you to relax consciously and release tension, anxiety, and troubling concerns when the lights go out. The basis of this method is a simple mental discipline of refusing to worry about *anything* in bed, including if or when you will go to sleep. You choose instead to practice the following conscious, progressive, deep relaxation method. And you return to it anytime you find that you have slipped back into *susto*. You discipline your attention by focusing it in somatic awareness on specific "anchors." This allows you to enter progressively deeper states of relaxation.

As with any learned skill, the "relaxation response" becomes ingrained in your neural pathways. You can begin to practice it in your daily life, consciously relaxing under pressure and releasing stress. The more you practice, both at night lying down and in the daytime in real-life situations, the more old stress-based habit patterns and reactions will gradually dissolve and be replaced by a new sustainable habit of conscious relaxation in response to stress.

How to Get Started

Practice the following exercise for twenty to thirty minutes per night for a period of at least one month and you will notice significant results besides the curing of your insomnia.

First, lie down on your back with your arms at your sides. Do not cross your legs. This position allows full relaxation, whereas if you lie on your side or cross your legs, the pressure on the body prevents full relaxation and the position itself is less conducive to maintaining clear awareness. In this position, do the basic Four-Step Shift:

Step One: Stop . . . Feel . . . Observe (unplug from the *susto* self)
Step Two: Relax Your Physical/Feeling Circuits (surrender your body into the ocean of Spirit energy)
Step Three: Relax Your Mental/Emotional Circuits (surrender your mind and emotions into the ocean of Spirit energy)
Step Four: Plug into the Web of Life (come alive in interdependence)

If you've been practicing the Four-Step Shift, you should be able to enter a state of deep, relaxed somatic awareness in two minutes.

If you haven't been practicing, you may want to reread the full exercise from Chapter Four before continuing. After doing these four steps, affirm the new bedtime-is-relaxation-mastery-time context from "Cognitive Reframing" on page 180. Feel it in your whole body, see the wisdom of it, and choose it as your purpose. Feel the shift that happens when you have truly made this commitment in somatic awareness.

The next part of this exercise is the classic whole-body deep-relaxation method. There is no substitute for learning this method. It allows you to enter profound states of deep, relaxed, somatic awareness at will. Starting with your feet, you are going to tense groups of muscles by turn for three seconds, then release the tension and focus on the sensation of the muscles relaxing. The initial tension, then the release, followed by intent focus on relaxation allows a deeper level of conscious physical relaxation to be attained than if you were simply to relax without prior conscious tensing of the muscles.

Do this initial tension/relaxation exercise with one muscle group at a time—i.e., first the left foot, then the right foot, left calf and shin, right calf and shin, left knee, right knee, left thigh, right thigh, left buttock, right buttock, stomach, back, chest, left hand, right hand, left forearm, right forearm, left bicep, right bicep, left shoulder, right shoulder, front of neck, back of neck, jaw, face, and finally the entire head.

Or you can do the muscles in "twin groups"—i.e., both feet, both calves and shins, both knees, both thighs, both buttocks, etc. Once you've completed the entire sequence, go into the process in "The Journey Down" described on page 184. (After two weeks of practicing this detailed tension/relaxation sequence followed by the Journey Down, your body will have learned the "relaxation response." Then you can tense and relax the entire body all at once, three times in succession, holding for three seconds of tension each time followed by ten seconds of conscious relaxation, except for the third time, when you will go into the total progressive relaxation of the Journey Down.)

The Journey Down

Having done the above tension/relaxation exercises, you should feel very relaxed. Now take a long, slow, complete breath and hold it in for ten to twenty seconds, focusing on the sense of deepening relaxation. Don't strain to hold the breath. Exhale it when it feels right, consciously releasing all restlessness, tension, or anxiety with the breath. Do three (or more) complete breaths in this way. After your last exhalation, scan your body with feeling attention, from head to toe. Practice relaxing and releasing any remaining tension or unease you notice in any part of your body. Do this scanning periodically throughout the exercise. It will deepen the progressive relaxation by keeping your attention anchored in the body via somatic awareness.

You should now be in a state of pronounced relaxation that feels very pleasant, even pleasurable. Take a minute or two to feel and savor this sensation. You may notice a gentle, sensual pulsing or tingling throughout your body. You may feel a sense of calm or peace. Savor them and let them penetrate every cell of your body.

Now it's time to go deeper. There are four key anchors for your attention that will ensure a progressive deepening of this relaxed state. These anchors also allow you to release any thoughts or concerns that may spontaneously arise. You may use any or all of them in any combination, as long as it allows you to maintain a focus and continue your descent into deeper levels of relaxation. These anchors are:

- Visualization and/or counting backward
- The pleasant bodily sensations of deepening relaxation
- The point between the eyebrows
- The breath

Visualization/counting backward: Some people are good at visualizing. If you are, one of the following visualizations may help you to go deeper: Going down a long, winding circular stairway. Lying on your back in the ocean and descending slowly into its warm, beautiful depths. Floating on a raft going down a gentle river through a beautiful jungle. Many other scenarios can be used. Pick or create one that feels right for you. As you visualize, we also recommend counting slowly backward in your mind from 50 to 0, or 100 to 0. If you have trouble visualizing, simply counting backward while using other anchors for your attention, as described below, will still allow you to reach the deepest states of relaxation.

The body: The body and its sensations are another key anchor for attention. So as you count down and/or visualize, it is important to stay connected through somatic awareness to the bodily sensations of deepening relaxation. This makes the exercise pleasurable on a physical level. It deepens conscious relaxation. And it anchors your attention and calms your mind.

The point between the brows: As you do the above, it helps to try to keep your closed eyes fixed on the bridge of the nose between the brows. This helps to focus the mind and keep it from wandering into random thinking.

The breath: The feeling and sound of the breath coming in and going out like the tide offer another soothing anchor for your attention that deepens relaxation and keeps the mind from wandering. Whenever you notice that your mind has gone astray, simply return to the above anchors and continue your progressive relaxation.

Do this progressive relaxation using the anchors as needed, and simply feel and enjoy the results. You may notice interesting sensory and other phenomena as your consciousness shifts. Common experiences include gentle pulsing or tingling sensations throughout the body; a sense of time slowing down; a sense of being pleasantly immersed in thick liquid; a dreamlike feeling, which may include interesting sounds, flashes of hypnogogic imagery, mini-dreamlike sequences, spontaneous creative thoughts or insights, and more.

If you have a spiritual or religious orientation, silently repeating a mantra or short prayer is also a good anchor for your attention. But stay focused on the sensations of bodily relaxation. If you do this exercise nightly for four to six weeks, your insomnia should become a thing of the past. And a new and interesting world will have opened up within you that you may wish to continue exploring. After a month of practice you will be able to "switch on" deep relaxation in moments. Once your insomnia is gone you can practice this method to achieve mastery of deep somatic awareness, or shamanic consciousness.

At this level, the purpose of practicing this method is not falling asleep, but rather staying awake in "the depths." The following method will allow you to descend to the deepest levels of consciousness remaining conscious and aware, and without falling asleep. It is called the Arm Up Method.

The Arm Up Method

Begin in the relaxation position, lying on your back with arms at your side. Raise your right or left forearm at your side so that it's resting on the elbow and pointing at the ceiling. As you enter deeper states of relaxation, your arm serves as a gentle alarm. If you begin drifting off to sleep, it will start to fall, bringing you to awareness at that level of relaxation without waking you up fully. Each time you start to fall asleep, the arm will begin to fall and you will return to awareness at that level. Continue the process using the attention anchors, going deeper in somatic awareness. This method allows you to explore the fascinating inner world and to witness the levels between waking and sleeping that we all pass through each night without conscious awareness. With sufficient practice, you can achieve lucid dreaming using this method.

My co-author, Doug, has been experimenting with these deep relaxation/somatic awareness methods since 1976. Below, he describes some of his experiments in the first person to show how the basic skill of deep relaxation can be applied in different ways and in different areas of life.

Doug: "I first learned the standard deep-relaxation method presented above with several refinements in a book on self-hypnosis. My intention at the time was to use self-hypnosis to improve my tennis game. The first thing I noticed was the sheer pleasure of deep relaxation. The second thing I noticed was the interesting altered states it produced. I was hooked! At that time I had suffered from chronic insomnia for five years, and it took me two to four hours to get to sleep each night. I had gotten used to my insomnia and had grudgingly accepted it as a permanent though unwelcome condition. To my surprise and relief, in less than a month of practicing the deep-relaxation method, my insomnia disappeared—an unintended and unexpected side effect. It has never returned. Since then I have been able to fall asleep almost at will, anywhere, at any time.

"I continued this practice because it was so pleasurable and so fascinating. With my newfound ability to relax, my tennis game, my temper, and my outlook on life noticeably improved. A year or so later I began writing seriously. Each night I would enter into the deep-relaxation state, where I would intentionally try to come up with creative ideas for stories. It worked beautifully. Not long after that I discovered the Arm Up technique in a book. This allowed me to go even deeper without falling asleep. I experienced various fascinating phenomena, including lucid dreaming.

"Two years into this intriguing practice, I took up meditation. I soon began to combine meditation techniques with my deep-relaxation practice, incorporating the anchors of the breath, the focus on the third eye, and the use of a mantra. Later I substituted contemplative prayer for the mantra, which often led to remarkable spiritual insights and dreams.

"Two specific applications of this deep-relaxation method are worth mentioning. In 1995 I was completing a book under contract with a publisher while working a forty-hour-a-week office job. The publisher's deadline was six weeks away. For those six weeks I worked forty hours a week at my job. I also worked at least forty-eight hours a week on the book. With commute time, meals, etc., I averaged one and a half to three hours' sleep a night for those six weeks. (Though one day each weekend I would sleep for ten hours.)

"Every night I lay down, did the Arm Up technique, and went into deep relaxation. Many nights I never put my arm down and never fell asleep. I simply remained in the pleasurable, rejuvenating, often profound states of deep relaxation until it was time to get up and go to work. It felt like being in suspended animation. One of the most fascinating aspects of this was the consistent time distortion I experienced. It always seemed as if many hours passed in those states. I would open my eyes three or four times each night, thinking that my two or three hours was over and it was time to get up. But each time I would find that what seemed like hours was no more than twenty or thirty minutes. I always got up feeling refreshed and energized, even if I hadn't fallen asleep. The state of conscious, deep relaxation seemed to be as refreshing as ordinary sleep itself.

"The second story shows how this deep relaxation method can be applied to releasing stress and functioning under pressure. In 1996 I applied for a job as a salesperson for a highly respected national reading and study-skills program. I had never done sales before, and was hired mainly because of my passion for reading, writing, and studying. It turned out to be an extremely high-pressure sales job. I worked in a room with seventy other salespeople, most of them experienced professionals. We each took twenty to thirty phone calls a day, with a few minutes in between each call. The work was commission based, meaning no sales, no paycheck, no job. The job was also seasonal and the number of calls coming in dwindled as the season progressed. Halfway through the season the company would begin letting people go. At the end, there would only be seven people left. We all knew this from the start.

"But when the firing started, a slaughterhouse feeling crept into the salesroom. One by one, people would be called into the office to see the boss, the blinds in his office would be drawn shut, and minutes later the unfortunate salesperson would emerge, get his or her things from his or her desk, say good-bye to friends, and go home. On breaks and during lunch, people would gather in small groups speculating on who would be let go next and who had a chance of being kept on. As the tension mounted, people grew increasingly anxious, more irritable with each other. Some people literally began to snap. I heard a few salespeople argue with, and even curse at, potential customers, sometimes angrily ending the calls by slamming the phone down. Some salespeople were let go for this behavior, which was essentially due to their inability to handle stress.

"I was an inexperienced salesperson. But I recognized the environment of fear, and I used the relaxation method for the several minutes in between sales calls. On my breaks, I went outside and did ten minutes of complete breathing followed by ten minutes of deep relaxation and meditation. On my lunch break I did some brief stretching and took a half-hour nap. I kept myself properly hydrated from the large water bottle on my desk.

"I was able to stay calm, relaxed, and clear for the entire season, while many of the more experienced salespeople were stressing out, sometimes acting out, and in some cases breaking down under pressure. I ended up making it to the final seven salespeople, and I was asked to stay on as part of the staff when the sales season ended. When I asked my supervisor why I had been kept on, he said it was because I remained calm, cheerful, and cooperative under pressure, and they preferred someone with those qualities to someone with better sales stats who lacked them.

"Mastery of the deep-relaxation method is perhaps the most important skill that I possess. It informs and supports every aspect of my life and is a significant factor in my consistent good health, positive outlook, and high energy level."

Insomnia Checklist: Dos and Don'ts

• Eliminate wakeful activities in bed, such as reading, working, watching TV, *and worrying*. Declare your bed a relaxation and sleep zone instead of a work and worry zone. You don't need to eliminate sexual activity from the bedroom. (Whew!)

• Monitor your caffeine, sugar, nicotine, alcohol, or drug intake. All of these can aggravate insomnia. None will help it. (Drugging or drinking yourself to sleep is no cure.)

• Check with your physician or pharmacist if you are taking any medications; they may have the side effect of insomnia.

• Get regular exercise. Studies show that non-exercisers have higher rates of insomnia than exercisers. Non-exercisers have cured insomnia through taking up a regular exercise program.

• Getting half an hour minimum of sunlight a day will help you sleep.

• Do several minutes of light stretching before going to bed.

• A twenty-minute walk after dinner followed by a hot bath or shower before bed is an excellent relaxation method.

• If the room is too warm it can prevent you from falling asleep.

• If there is light or noise coming into your bedroom, you may want to try an eye pillow and earmuffs. Very comfortable and effective earmuffs used for firing ranges can be purchased at most sporting-goods stores.

• Afternoon naps improve sleep and daily functioning. Avoid the tendency to override the typical afternoon energy lag with artificial stimulants such as caffeine, sweets, or cigarettes. If you can't nap at work, use your break time to do some stretching, deep breathing, and meditation or relaxation.

• Practice this deep-relaxation method in the afternoon whenever possible. Ten minutes is sufficient; thirty minutes is a luxury. Practicing after any kind of exercise allows you to go easily to deeper levels.

• Commit to practicing the method every night for one month just before sleep.

• Remember, you're not trying to go to sleep. Don't make sleep the focus. Make your deepening relaxation through the method the focus.

• Practice this relaxation response at random moments during the day to anchor it as a response to stress.

• Intentionally practice relaxing in the face of stress until it becomes a reliable skill. It will give you a new confidence in life.

• Also practice in the face of anxiety, depression, or any other stress-based emotional or psychological ailment. You will realize the same satisfaction and confidence as you see positive, healing results in these areas. The more you do this, the more stress will become a signal to relax, to shift into your sustainable self, and to access the varied inner resources that allow you to impact people and situations positively.

• Finally, poor functioning or unhealthy habits in other gateways—a bad diet, insufficient exercise, poor hydration and oxygenation, overwork, and more—can cause or contribute to insomnia, directly and indirectly. So assess your functioning in these and other gateways and begin to make healthy changes. The self-assessment questionnaire in Chapter Seventeen, "Nature's Energy Medicine Chest," will help you do this.

15
Sexuality: Curing Sexual Dysfunction through Sensual Communion

Sex, the primal instinctive drive that originally ensured the survival of our species, has become the dominating obsession and primary marketing tool of Western culture. This most intimate expression of love between two people is evoked to sell thousands of products from soft drinks, cigarettes, and alcohol to toothpaste, guns, and automobiles. Daily, from every media and venue, our minds and libidos are shrewdly stimulated and manipulated with provocative, titillating sexual imagery and messages. We are trained, subliminally and overtly, to model and measure our personalities, behavior, physical appearance, and even our relationships by arbitrary and artificial ideas, standards, and images that tell us what is, and why we need to be, "sexy."

Our culture's obsession with and mass marketing of sex have created mass confusion and distorted ideas about the nature and healthy expression of sexuality. Popular culture equates being "sexy" with seduction, manipulation, power, conquest, and even adultery. Sex (or being sexy) is the implied solution to loneliness, boredom, depression, lack of purpose, poverty, low self-esteem, and more. This false advertising, which is psychologically manipulative, is harmful at an individual and a cultural level.

Sex is not a solution to anything. Its most basic purposes are procreation, expressing love, deepening emotional and spiritual intimacy, and conducting spirit energy. We instinctively yearn for profound intimacy, to be seen, known, accepted, and loved as we are. Through sex, this can occur in the deepest possible way. And when this innate need is not fulfilled in our sexual relationships, they become a source of stress.

Yet if sex is not a solution to anything, numerous scientific studies have shown that sex provides many health benefits. Some are listed below.

• Men who have sex three times a week reduce the risk of heart attacks and strokes by 50 percent. Sex also increases testosterone and is good for the prostate gland.

• Having sex once a week or more boosts the immune system, increasing our ability to fight off illness.

• Regular sex for women triggers an increase in female hormones, keeps the vaginal tract healthy, and lowers the risk of heart disease.

• An average session of sex consumes 200 calories. This is equivalent to a fifteen-minute run on a treadmill.

• Sexual activity strengthens bones and muscles.

• Sexual intimacy lowers anxiety and reduces depression.

• Sex and orgasm dramatically increase the hormone oxytocin, which triggers the release of painkilling endorphins. Sex can bring pain relief to a variety of conditions, from arthritis to migraines to PMS.

• Sex increases oxygenation of the cells and stimulates improved functioning of most organs and the circulatory systems in the body.

• According to a study of 3,500 men and women between the

ages of 18 and 102, conducted by clinical neuropsychologist Dr. David Weeks of Scotland's Royal Edinburgh Hospital, *regular sex retards the aging process!*

The Power of Eros

The above health benefits are not surprising when we consider that through sex, we conduct the primal power of Eros. Eros drives the instinctive "urge to merge," the instinct for love, orgasm, and procreation. It drives the urge to create, to know deeply, to make one's mark in the world. And it drives the desires for ego transcendence, enlightenment, spiritual freedom, and union with God.

And it is more than that. Eros is the vital, attractive, creative, and destructive force continually erupting in all of nature, impregnating, germinating and blossoming, ripening, rotting and decaying, devouring, digesting and recycling all things into new life. It drives the jungle's seething fecundity and the hurricane's fury. It draws atoms together to create matter, and draws living creatures to merge in sexual union. It is the intoxicating, nonrational intensity in love, desire, orgasm, agony, rage, and even madness. It is found in the convulsive pangs of birth and death. It is the mysterious drive in every plant straining toward sunlight; in every newborn creature yearning for its mother; in every soul longing for God. Its most archetypal expression is the Big Bang that gave birth to the universe.

Human sexuality is a minor emanation of universal Eros. Yet we humans struggle with sex as a primal force, and as a moral and social issue, because it threatens to bind us to our animal nature, to erotic desire and procreation, and because, on some level, we both fear and crave this bondage.

Eros, as a higher spiritual drive, may lead us into religious, mystical, or shamanic paths. Yet its higher calling can also be fulfilled through our sexuality. Countless ordinary people have, during sex, spontaneously experienced profound, even life-changing altered states of consciousness that parallel those of classical mystical and religious experiences.

Yet despite the latent higher potentials and earthly pleasures in sex, most of us get bogged down in its lower realms. Sex is both a source of stress and a casualty of stress for millions of Americans. It is more often a source of uncertainty, anxiety, confusion, and pain than a source of ecstatic union. Sexual problems, dysfunctions, and obsessions are epidemic in our culture.

Susto and Sex

Most sexual dysfunctions are not of physical origins. They are stress based, or psychosomatic, rather than physical. They are rooted in *susto*. They originate in the mind and emotions in response to formative, often wounding experiences and relationships. And they typically involve negative beliefs about sex, fears of sexual inadequacy or failure, fears of sexual contact, or fears of being open, vulnerable, and intimate with another person. Common sexual problems include the loss of libido, inability to have an erection or achieve orgasm, and a variety of sexual compulsions, perversions, and addictions.

The most common sexual problems for men are sexual performance anxiety, erectile dysfunction, and premature ejaculation. They are often linked. The most common sexual problems for women are anorgasmia, or the inability to achieve orgasm, and vaginismus, an involuntary contraction of the vaginal muscles that makes intercourse impossible. (Both could be called female sexual performance anxiety.) The most common sexual problems for couples are poor communication and intimacy skills, not knowing how to relax and be fully present, and a lack of trust or deep intimacy in the relationship and therefore in bed. And each partner bringing his or her unique "hang-ups" into the relationship further complicates the relationship and compromises the sex.

When Viagra burst onto the scene, many men, and many couples, thought their sexual problems were solved. The magic blue pill that guaranteed an erection that made the sexual act mechanically possible seemed like chemical magic. But the new sexual wonder drugs do not manufacture passion, increase energy, heal relationship problems, emotional wounds and sexual compulsions, or resolve the emotional, psychological, or physical issues that underlie most sexual dysfunctions. Nor do they open the door to the profound emotional and sexual communion that is one of the deepest human needs and the basis of great sex. The new drugs have benefited many, but many have also learned that you don't heal the roots just by stiffening the branches.

Most sexual problems and dysfunctions can be healed in time through healthy relationships to the energy gateways. But the ability to shift into our sustainable self in intimate relationship is what primarily heals sexual anxiety or dysfunction. It also allows us to experience profound emotional and sexual communion and a mutually satisfying sex life.

Let's briefly examine the roots of sexual dysfunctions.

Performance Pressures and Root Problems

Men and women feel sexual anxiety, and develop sexual dysfunctions, for varied reasons. There are often specific causes, like overwork, chronic stress, or unresolved business or relationship problems. Unrealistic and nonrelational expectations, attitudes, and behaviors regarding sex promoted in the culture at large also contribute to sexual anxiety and confusion. Movies, TV shows, advertisements, and commercials all prey on our sexual insecurities, making us feel unattractive or inadequate. Image, status, performance, technique, and orgasm are overemphasized, while trust, presence, awareness, and intimacy are underrated or ignored.

Popular culture encourages us to rush into sex for misguided reasons, before intimacy and trust have been established. This approach reduces sex to a mere quest for pleasure and orgasm, which is like masturbation, or to a quest for self-esteem, glamour, or prestige, which reduces sex to ego masturbation. But satisfying sexual intimacy is not achieved through techniques that produce only orgasm. Trust, openness, somatic awareness, and presence are also required. Without these, sex becomes mechanical and inherently stressful. Our spirit desires intimacy and presence as much as our body desires sexual pleasure. Great sex, satisfying sex, healing sex, emerges naturally out of deep intimacy.

Modern psychology traces the roots of much sexual anxiety and compulsion to confusing, painful, or traumatic experiences and family dynamics, often going back to childhood. Contributing factors may include sexual trauma from molestation to rape; emotional or physical abuse; sexually repressed or promiscuous family environments; unhealthy or unhappy relationships between parents, and/or between parents and children; negative religious and secular attitudes and teachings about sex and the body; and more. All these shape our beliefs and ideas about sex, the body, and our masculine and feminine identities and roles and affect our capacity for emotional and sexual intimacy.

Because of its roots in pain or trauma, the *susto* self instinctively and self-protectively recoils from deep intimacy and vulnerability. And we are never more exposed and vulnerable than when naked in bed with a lover who is watching us, intimately pressed against us, full of his or her own desires, hopes, fears, self-doubts, confusion, and unhealed emotional and sexual wounds. In sexual performance anxiety, a lover has become an audience we fear to fail, disappoint, or displease. And *susto* is directing the show.

Fortunately, we don't have to heal all our emotional and psychological wounds to experience a deep and healing emotional and sexual intimacy. Our ability to shift into our sustainable self is the key to sustainable sex and to the healing of many sexual dysfunctions. Feeling awareness, presence, curiosity, openness, vulnerability, and trust are an innate part of who we are. These qualities of the sustainable self make profound intimacy possible. And this intimacy is what we long for in life, in friendships, and in sex, whether we know it or not, even if it's also what we fear.

Sustainable Intimacy, Sustainable Sex

Sexual dysfunctions are similar to insomnia. Both are stress-related disorders in which fears and debilitating thoughts become a habitual or compulsive focus of attention in relation to a specific function— sleep or sex. In both dysfunctions these fears and thoughts become a primary focus at the most inopportune time, virtually creating the feared result.

The cure for most sexual dysfunctions, like the cure for insomnia, begins with cognitive reframing. You recognize your current anxiety-producing perspectives and fears and exchange them for positive, reassuring, even inspiring perspectives and knowledge. This requires some mental discipline, but it is not merely a mental process. It is done by adapting the Four-Step Shift to an intimate emotional and sexual encounter.

The first step is recognizing the psychosomatic nature of the sexual dysfunction, and to know that it can be healed. And while

ENERGY AND LIBIDO CHECKLIST

It is important to remember that negative habits in other gateways—bad diet, under-oxygenation or under-hydration, lack of exercise, insomnia, chronic tension, an inability to relax and release stress, substance abuse, and more—can distort our thinking, perceiving, and emotions and diminish our energy and our sex drive. In Chapter Seventeen, "Nature's Medicine Chest," you can assess your sexual energy and issues in relation to your "performance" in the other gateways.

the roots of any sexual dysfunction may lie in formative relationships, traumas, or environments, *it is always being unintentionally or compulsively stimulated in the present in the mind.* A sexual dysfunction is really a habit of attention that triggers uncomfortable or unwanted feelings or undesired physical effects. And that habit can be changed.

The second step is to reframe the purpose of the intimate time you spend with your lover. It also helps if your lover or partner knows what you want to do, and why. The new healing context for intimate time is different than what is conventionally expected in bed. It directly involves your partner, and real intimacy depends upon your fully including him or her. Your partner's support and understanding will also significantly and positively affect the outcome.

Here is our recommendation for reframing your intimate time with your lover. In conventional sex, the "goal" is pleasure and orgasm. But here there is no goal. Intimate time is now time to relax, physically and emotionally, with your partner; to be fully present emotionally and sensually; to be curious and explore a lover with your eyes and through touch; to deepen intimacy and to see where it leads and what is revealed. And to enjoy every part of the experience.

We recommend that you do this exercise with your partner for at least one hour three times a week. It should be done after a bath or shower, in bed or in some other comfortable location, when there are no pressing time constraints.

Exploring Sustainable Intimacy

• Begin by putting on soft music.

• Simply be present, your attention on your partner, and also be anchored in somatic awareness. You are doing a version of the Four-Step Shift, only now with your partner as an additional focus of attention.

• Be curious. Look into your partner's eyes. Who is this person, in *this* moment, looking at you? Feel the mystery and the presence of the being looking out of those eyes.

• Slowly, gently, with feeling awareness, explore your partner's body, face, all over, with your hands. (You can also use your feet.) Notice other places where your bodies touch. There is no right or wrong. Don't try to please. Simply feel, be aware, be present. Express without thought, a motive, a goal.

• Continually release all thoughts, all concerns, all expectations. Do this by focusing on feeling and observing. This emotional and sensory awareness is the beginning and the foundation of emotional and sexual communion.

• Express what you feel through touch, through looks, through your breath, with sounds. Express affection, desire, curiosity, delight, without words.

• Do this exploration for at least half an hour, or more.

• For the last part of this exercise, simply stare deeply into each other's eyes for ten to fifteen minutes. You can hold each other as you do this, but be still. Simply feel, relax, breathe naturally, notice and release all thoughts that come, while surrendering into your partner's eyes and into his or her presence.

This basic exercise is useful in healing almost any emotional and sexual dysfunction. It also develops and deepens intimacy and trust that make profound emotional and sexual communion possible. Do this exercise three times a week for at least two weeks before having intercourse. Don't rush. Give this process time. Be present, be curious, explore, express, be aware, and discover what happens.

When you begin to have intercourse, continue to apply the same process exactly as described above for at least two weeks. Avoid coming to orgasm for the hour or so of the exercise. This may mean periodic or even prolonged periods of stillness. But if you are doing the exercise above, it will be a dynamic stillness full of deep sensory and emotional awareness.

Notice if you find yourself slipping back into an old mind-set, worried about performing, trying to please, etc. Talk with your partner during, or after, if there is something you want to communicate or want to understand. At this point, with intimacy established, communication and coaching between you about what feels good or doesn't feel good are fine. Trust and intimate communication in bed are also "sexy."

A Case Study

When Frank, a thirty-two-year-old carpenter, met Linda, a twenty-six-year-old bookkeeper, he hadn't been in a relationship, and hadn't had sex, for several years. He had, in previous relationships, suffered from sexual performance anxiety and premature ejaculation. After dating for a few weeks, he and Linda became more serious. And Frank began to feel anxious about being unable to "perform" and satisfy Linda sexually.

When they finally went to bed, Frank was unable to have an erection. Linda was fine about it. She knew the basics of the sustainable-intimacy exercise above. She told Frank not to worry about having sex. She explained the intimacy exercise to Frank and they practiced it together. Both of them found it extremely intimate and satisfying.

They did this exercise more than three times a week for several weeks. In that time, Frank was unable to achieve an erection. With Linda's support, he didn't worry about it. "It will happen when we're ready," she told him. And it did, quite naturally. After that, they continued practicing the exercise, now with intercourse. They are now married. And their intimacy and their sex life are mutually satisfying.

Frank and Linda both agree that the period before Frank achieved an erection allowed them to explore each other in a unique way, and to establish a remarkable intimacy, without the stress and pressure of performance anxiety that both men and women tend to experience in the early phase of a sexual relationship. "They were," says Frank, "three of the most intimate and beautiful weeks of our relationship." Frank also believes that without the sustainable-intimacy exercise, his anxiety about being unable to have an erection might have turned it into a chronic condition.

This chapter is not comprehensive. If you feel you have a serious emotional or psychological problem that requires greater help, we recommend that you consult with a therapist who deals with sexual issues. If you have a physically based sexual problem, we recommend that you consult a physician, though the above exercise is still highly beneficial. We also recommend that you read other books on the subject of sexuality and sexual dysfunction for greater understanding. There are many good ones.

16

Addiction: The Craving for Spirit and the Shift to a Sustainable Self

addiction: any compulsive, isolating, unhealthy dependence on a substance, person, behavior, or activity, usually driven by fear, pain, and spiritual emptiness

Shamans say the soul seeks periodic release from the stressful confines of the *susto* self, a release into a greater life and consciousness through healing communion with Spirit. Psychologists tell us that humans (and other animals) instinctively and periodically crave altered states of consciousness, seeking temporary relief from the pressures of life. Anthropologists recognize this innate need for periodic release from ordinary self-consciousness as the basis of the social and ceremonial use of intoxicating substances in all cultures. Alcohol, tea, tobacco, marijuana, and numerous other natural "mind-altering drugs" were all originally used as sacraments in religious rituals. Shamanism itself was born out of man's earliest encounters with such mind-altering substances.

This innate need to change our consciousness is also the basis of "mind-altering" spiritual disciplines like meditation, prayer, yoga, and chanting. It gave rise to original forms of "sacred theater" like ritual dance, music, song, and storytelling. (Even modern forms of popular entertainment may serve this higher purpose.) The hope behind all such ceremonies, rituals, and sacraments is that, through a change in consciousness, we will be fundamentally and spiritually changed or healed in some way.

But there has always been an unhealthy shadow side to this need to change our state. The need for stimulation and release can become an unhealthy craving or obsession that undermines our relationships, our normal, healthy functioning, and our well-being. When this happens, we have entered the realm of addiction.

The widespread phenomenon of addiction affects our lives and our culture in countless ways. Alcoholism is the most prevalent and destructive addiction on the planet. In America there are an estimated 14 million adult alcoholics. An estimated 3 million teenagers from ages fourteen to seventeen have a drinking problem. An estimated 76 million adults have an alcoholic in the family by birth or by marriage.

The combined costs of alcohol and drug abuse in America total $250 billion to $300 billion annually. Alcohol is a known factor in 100,000 deaths per year, and an unknown factor in many more. (This includes 41 percent of all traffic fatalities.) The combined statistics for all addictions—to alcohol, to cigarettes, to illegal and prescription drugs, to gambling, to food, to sex, to unhealthy relationships, to high-risk behaviors, to work, to shopping, and more—are unknown. And their costs in money, in human pain, in unfulfilled potential, and in devastated lives are incalculable.

A Shamanic View of Addiction

Shamans view addiction as an extreme expression of *susto*, a desperate effort to escape the fear, pain, and loneliness of our disconnection from Spirit. The root of addiction is an innate hunger for healing contact with Spirit, and the behaviors of addiction are a distorted quest for that healing contact.

Shamans also see *susto* as the primary addiction of human life. *Susto* is an addiction to fear that separates us from our indigenous self, from Spirit, and blocks the flow of spirit energy in us. In *susto*, we habitually or compulsively "ingest" toxic, fear-based thoughts and feelings that immediately skew our perceptions and alter our consciousness. This depletes our energy, undermines our health, and diminishes the quality of our lives over time. As we have shown in previous chapters, *susto* is at the root of most of the dysfunctional patterns that manifest in the gateways, and this includes all addictions.

Therefore, shamans see addiction as a spiritual illness as well as a biochemical one. And as with anxiety and depression, its healing necessarily requires a shift in consciousness that opens us to a direct encounter with Spirit, the power that heals, and a change of life habits in the gateways through simple disciplines that support our healing.

Bill Wilson: Modern Shaman, Healer of Addictions

Bill Wilson founded Alcoholics Anonymous after being healed of alcoholism through a profound experience of Spirit. Prior to his remarkable transformation, he had struggled desperately for years to give up alcohol but he was continually overpowered by his addiction.

The turning point came when he had lost all hope. His health ruined, diagnosed with brain damage from years of heavy drinking, his life and marriage in a shambles, and still unable to stop drinking,

Bill fell into a suicidal depression. He retreated to his room and began what he knew and half hoped would be a last binge ending in his death.

In the course of this binge, Ebbie, an old drinking buddy, stopped by to tell Bill that God had cured him of his alcoholism. God, Ebbie said, could cure Bill, too. All Bill had to do was pray and surrender his life to Him. Bill was impressed by his friend's apparent cure. But he was an atheist. And when Ebbie left he continued drinking. But a seed was planted. One day not long after, in his utter desperation, Bill cried out for God to show Himself, if He existed.

"Suddenly," he writes, "my room blazed with an indescribably white light. I was seized with an ecstasy beyond description. Every joy I had known was pale by comparison. . . . I was conscious of nothing else for a time. Then there was a great mountain. I stood upon its summit where a great wind blew. A wind not of air, but of spirit. In great, clean strength, it blew right through me. Then came the blazing thought, 'You are a free man.' I became acutely conscious of a Presence, a veritable sea of living spirit. I lay on the shores of a new world; I seemed possessed by the absolute, and the curious conviction that no matter how wrong things seemed to be, there could be no question of the ultimate rightness of God's universe. . . . For the first time I felt that I really belonged. I knew that I was loved and could love in return."

Bill Wilson returned to ordinary consciousness and he never took another drink. But he still wrestled with the compulsion to drink. Soon after, he realized that he needed to seek out and help other alcoholics who were struggling with their addictions in order to deepen his own process of healing and transformation. He incorporated this altruistic principle into AA early on. Soon after this realization, he and another recovered alcoholic, Robert Smith, started the first AA meetings.

From the beginning AA stressed that an addict's recovery required the help of, and ongoing contact with, "a higher power," accessed through prayer.

Like a true shaman, Bill Wilson was healed by a life-transforming encounter with Spirit. And he spent the rest of his life helping others to be healed of their addictions by continually choosing to seek the help of "a higher power" while progressively engaging in healing disciplines in the gateways through the Twelve Steps.

Since the late 1930s, hundreds of millions of alcoholics and addicts around the world have beaten their addictions by accessing the same Spirit that healed Bill Wilson, and by conducting spirit energy in their lives through the disciplines known as the Twelve Steps. AA is the most successful program on the planet for treating addiction. The reason for this is that it incorporates proactive disciplines in several key gateways that bring about a spiritual transformation of character. And it leads addicts to create a new life on the basis of that transformation, and on the principles that sustain it. These gateways are:

The Mind/Soul Gateway: AA members are encouraged to seek daily the help and guidance of a "higher power" for their healing. They are also encouraged to examine their thoughts, motives, and actions and strive to overcome character defects like anger, resentment, selfishness, and self-pity—all with the help of a higher power.

The Relationship Gateway: AA members ground their healing process in human relationships, with a high value placed on honesty, integrity, and accountability within the Twelve-Step process. They attend regular meetings where they learn to communicate honestly about their illness and their recovery process, with all its ups and downs. All new members have a personal sponsor with whom they are in regular contact, and with whom they develop a relationship based in honesty and trust. A truthful relationship to self is also developed through AA's rigorous and ongoing practical, ethical, and moral self-examination. When they are ready, AA members begin to clean up personal messes, resolve conflicts, make apologies, and redress wrongs they have previously done to others. All of these principles of "right relationship" are recognized as integral components of the healing process. And they work.

The Sustainable Reciprocity Gateway: All AA members at some point engage in ongoing altruistic action by becoming a sponsor to one or more new members. Helping others is recognized as a key component in the healing process, and AA members are encouraged to do so any time they find themselves struggling with temptation. Bill Wilson called this principle of healing through helping others "passing it on."

AA's success rate in helping addicts break free of their addictions is truly extraordinary, especially considering the fact that no drugs or medicines or personally supervised therapy are used in weaning addicts of their self-destructive compulsions and dependencies. AA does not promise radiant vitality and health to its members, nor does it teach the proactive disciplines in the gateways that produce vitality and health. It is a program for getting and staying sober one day at a time, with the help of a higher power and the support of the Twelve Steps and the AA community.

Healing Is More Than a Cessation of Symptoms

There is a gateway to a higher power, to Spirit, within each of us. As we discussed in Chapter Thirteen, "Depression," when we choose Spirit in our spirit, that power comes into us to do works of healing and transformation. Countless individuals have been healed of every imaginable affliction by the intervention of Spirit. But many of us do not choose Spirit until we are desperate, when our inner resources are depleted and our life as we have known and lived it has failed.

The choice for and the intervention of Spirit, and the awakening it triggers, is the essence of all spiritual paths, including the shamanic path. It is also essential for the genuine healing of spiritual afflictions like depression, anxiety, and addiction. But our full healing, which includes our continuing vitality and health, requires us to take responsibility for our habits and behaviors in the gateways.

The following two stories demonstrate the healing of addiction in two very different people in very different ways. Both involve the intervention of Spirit, and a new life established on its basis in the gateways.

The Healing of a Hard-Core Addiction

Paul, an Irishman in his early seventies, is a former heroin addict who has been "clean" for nearly forty years. He began using heroin in Dublin in his early twenties. It soon developed into a daily habit. Within a few years, his addiction completely ruled his life. As he couldn't hold down a real job, to support his habit he became a self-employed petty thief, burglar, and an occasional begger of money from friends, acquaintances, and strangers. His own family broke off relations with him because he kept stealing things from them to sell in order to buy heroin.

By the time Paul was thirty, he had made many attempts to stop using. All of them had failed. He had tried quitting "cold turkey" and he had tried working with a local drug-rehab program. He always succumbed to the overwhelming pull of his addiction and began using again, usually within a few weeks.

He grew more desperate, depressed, and hopeless as years passed. He began to contemplate suicide, which seemed an increasingly attractive option compared to the degradation in which he lived. What he calls "the change" happened when he was thirty-three.

"I was squatting in an abandoned building that served as a free hotel for local junkies," he reports. "I was extremely ill, lying on a dirty mattress in a little room on the second floor, unable to go out and steal anything to sell for a fix. Then withdrawal set in. I lay there shaking in agony all day, alone, thinking about my life. I felt utterly hopeless. I wanted to die and have it be over. I remember saying over and over, 'Please, God, get me out of here. I don't want to live like this.'

"I was in a kind of delirium. I felt death very near me. And I was completely willing to die. Early that evening I started fading in and out of consciousness. And at some point, I felt myself leave my body and shoot out into space at incredible speed, into a field of light that was indescribable. It was pure light, pure love, pure spirit. It was whatever God is. I don't know how long I stayed there. I was floating in a womblike bliss, being loved like I had never been loved. I knew everything was good, and always had been. Everything was all right."

At some point, Paul found himself back in his body. He was weak, but the sickness had passed. In the coming days, he discovered that his craving for heroin had completely and mysteriously vanished. It never returned. His astonishing experience changed him. He immediately embarked on a spiritual quest that led him around the world and that continues to this day. He changed his life habits in many ways and became, in his own words, "a grateful, healthy, functioning member of the human race." He reports that he has been healthy, productive, and growing ever since.

The Healing of a Psychological Addiction

Roger started smoking pot at the age of thirteen, in the mid-1970s, getting stoned with friends on weekends. By the time he was fifteen he was getting stoned several times a week, drinking beer, and also using speed. At sixteen he was smoking pot up to several times a day, drinking beer once a week or more, and using speed and cocaine several times a month or more, often injecting it into his arm with a hypodermic syringe. He wasn't chemically addicted to drugs, but he was psychologically dependent on getting high, and he experienced strong anxiety if he went for a day without doing so.

Then his family moved to another town, a small town where drugs were hard to find. Roger brought enough marijuana with him to last for a few months, and he knew he could always find a way to get beer. His new house was a few blocks from a local basketball court. He began to go there after school and play basketball with the neighborhood crowd. It was fun, a great workout, and he found that he had a natural affinity for the game. He began to get more serious about it. When school ended, he spent the following summer almost entirely on the basketball court. He says he played at least four hours a day and sometimes more.

As his physical condition improved, and his love of the game increased, Roger began drinking and using drugs less. He got stoned once or twice a week, but he considered it recreational. The next year he made the school basketball team. A strict coach and a rigorous training regime kept his drug use in check. But he still reached for drugs or alcohol when the pressures of life built up in him.

Roger went on to play basketball at a small college. He also began to refine his diet and his exercise regime, to improve his fitness. And he began to experiment with meditation as a way to clear his mind, to "get that cutting edge" on the basketball court. He still smoked pot and drank beer a few times a month, when he felt he needed a break from the stresses of life. It seemed a reasonable stress outlet, a way to kick back and relax. He assumed that was just the way things were.

Then one day Roger had a profound experience during meditation. "I felt a spiritual presence literally descend into me from above," he recalls. "I experienced the deepest peace and joy I've ever known. It lasted for maybe half an hour. But it changed my whole perspective. Drugs and alcohol had never given me anything like it. I knew I had experienced God or Spirit, or whatever you want to call it. And I wanted more."

Within three months of this experience, Roger had completely sworn off drugs and alcohol and embarked on a serious and committed spiritual path that involved daily meditation and yoga practice, a vegetarian diet, and a variety of other healthy disciplines in the gateways. He's been pursuing this path ever since. And except for a glass of wine once a year at holiday dinners, he's never returned to drugs or alcohol. Today he is a happy, married, successful entrepreneur who does regular service in his community.

Paul and Roger's stories show how Spirit can intervene to play a significant, even a decisive, role in healing physical and psychological addictions. Shamans see Spirit intervention not just as a support in the healing of addictions, but as a necessity. They see addiction as a disease of the spirit whose healing requires a new, sustainable self infused with Spirit, and a new, sustainable life founded in healthy disciplines and habits in the gateways. Without this, the best an addict can hope for is a successful ongoing struggle to manage both his addiction and the unhealed compulsions that drive it.

If you are struggling with an addiction, whether to a substance or a behavior, we strongly recommend the AA work, which has been tested and proven over decades. Why fight this serious disease on your own, or try to reinvent the wheel when your life is at stake?

We also recommend that you apply the wisdom that shamans in every spiritual tradition have proclaimed, and call on Spirit to come into you to begin the work of healing, rebirth, and transformation. And we recommend that you apply the gateway disciplines presented in this book, which will provide enormous support in the healing of addiction.

You've learned enough in the previous chapters to know what changes you need to make and what support structures you need to develop in the various gateways. More importantly, you know how to shift into your indigenous self, release stress, and access Spirit. Now it's time to develop a clear, simple proactive plan that will give you the abundant energy, vitality, and health that define a sustainable self.

In the next chapter you will do exactly that. You will thoroughly investigate your habits in each gateway, in the light of any issue or ailment you may currently be dealing with. And you will write your own prescription for a Spirit-infused, energy-filled life.

Section Four

Nature's Energy Medicine Chest

17

Your Personal Prescription to Spirited Energy

Taking Responsibility for Energy Management

We are each responsible for our level of vitality and health. And we all want both to be optimum. But we aren't always willing to invest the energy that attaining them requires. Optimum vitality and health are a by-product of a life grounded in healthy, energy-efficient, energy-generating habits in the gateways.

There are three basic levels of responsibility for energy and health. In Level One, we are ignorant of or indifferent to energy and health principles and take little or no responsibility. We take the path of least resistance, and that path generally leads downhill sooner or later. We unthinkingly abdicate responsibility for our energy and health, passing it on at best to doctors or the health-care system.

In Level One we may not exercise, we may eat poorly, we may indulge in sweets, cigarettes, alcohol, or drugs. We have no interest in learning deep relaxation or meditation skills. Our physical habits especially tend to be undisciplined, enervating, and degenerative, and our inner life may suffer accordingly. And our lifestyle accelerates the process of enervation and decline into illness, old age, and death.

In Level Two we are aware of general health and energy principles. We do not grossly abuse our body and mind, nor do we assiduously devote ourselves to their care. We are generally moderate in our habits, and provide our body and mind with basic, responsible self-maintenance. We eat an average healthy Western diet, with periodic lapses. We may exercise periodically but perhaps not regularly.

We would like to be dynamically fit, healthy, and vital, but this just isn't high on our priority list. It takes too much effort and responsibility, and we lack sufficient energy and motivation. So we settle for average energy and health within our comfort zone. Still, compared to Level One, we are doing just fine. We view our limited energy, our periodic illnesses, and our occasional health crises as the normal toll of living. And as most of the population lives at this level, it does seem normal. But it's far below the radiant vitality and health we are designed for and could have with a little more effort.

Western medicine, with its remedial rather than proactive approach, colludes with these two levels, daily dispensing vast amounts of pharmaceuticals for ailments that could be cured through proactive living. Most of us have experienced these first two levels at different times in our lives. Fewer people progress to the third level, though more are doing so every year.

In Level Three we are knowledgeable in, or are learning about, health and energy principles. And we are proactively seeking vitality and health through disciplined habits and right living on the basis of these principles. But if our search for greater energy and health is *susto*-driven, then our "positive" health habits will also be linked to physical and emotional stress. Fanatical dietary, exercise, or other health practices that put unhealthy strain or stress on the body and mind tend to diminish somatic awareness. Such regimes may help you get fit and lose weight, and may provide other benefits. But if they are stressful to maintain in the present, they have unhealthy liabilities in the long run.

The ideal Level Three is wholly positive and sustainable in the long run. Many people do achieve optimum vitality and health through dynamic yet balanced participation in the gateways. They eat a healthy diet, get sufficient exercise, are meaningfully connected to life through their work and relationships, and regularly engage in some form of meditative or somatic awareness practice that allows them to relax, release stress, and achieve a measure of peace and joy in life.

The Gateway Evaluations

The following evaluation, presented in a series of questionnaires, will help you assess your habits and your level of responsibility in the gateways. Then it will help you make progressive, practical changes that support your shift into the vitality and health of the sustainable version of Level Three. Each questionnaire focuses on one gateway. It allows you to notice where you are bringing energy in, where you are neglecting to bring energy in, and where you are actively leaking energy in that gateway. At the end of each questionnaire you will write a simple proactive energy and health prescription for that gateway.

When you've completed all eight questionnaires, you will have an overview of your energy habits in these gateways. You may notice general patterns of behavior, both positive and negative, appearing in various gateways. And you will have written an overall energy and health prescription that includes all of the gateways and that is tailored to address your particular issues, conditions, and needs. This evaluation will give you a deeper understanding that, in itself, will release new energy and motivation for change.

We recommend that you answer the questions below on a notepad. As you do this evaluation, keep in mind any life, energy, or health issues you are currently dealing with. If you are struggling with anxiety, depression, an eating disorder, or a job or relationship problem, notice how your energy-depleting habits or leaks in various gateways may be connected to this unresolved condition and be adding stress to it. As you do each checklist, look for negative thoughts, beliefs, and emotions that underlie energy-depleting habits and behaviors. And if you have a serious medical or psychiatric condition, we recommend that you also consult a competent and open-minded physician.

Evaluations, Diagnoses, and Prescriptions for an Energy-Filled Life

The Food Entrada Checklist

• Is your diet generally healthy, with a daily balance of fresh and cooked foods, of fruits, vegetables, and proteins?
• Do you eat a lot of processed, starchy, or fatty foods high in sugar and salt?
• Do you eat only when you're hungry?
• Do you eat automatically by the clock whether you're hungry or not?
• Do you eat randomly in the day?
• Do you pay close attention to the feeling in your stomach before you eat or snack, to see if you're really hungry?
• How do you generally feel in the period after eating?

- Do you feel energized after a meal?
- Do you feel lethargic or sleepy after a meal?
- Do you eat or snack in response to nervousness, pressure, stress, or anxiety?
- Are you overweight? Underweight? If either, how much?
- Do you feel good about your dietary habits? (This includes your food choices, the amounts you eat per sitting or per snack, and the frequency of your eating.)
- Do you feel good about your energy level?
- Do you feel that you burn off the food you eat?
- On a scale of 1 to 10, rate the following food motivations as they apply to you: Eating for fuel and energy. Eating for convenience. Eating for emotional solace. Eating to suppress anxiety. Eating out of boredom. Eating for taste and pleasure.
- Based on all of the above answers, can you see any correlation between your current dietary habits and your current energy and health levels or problems?
- What is your idea of the ideal diet for you? Are you eating it now?

Assessment: Intuitively assess your current level of dietary energy efficiency, from 1 (a daily diet of pure junk food) to 10 (a perfect daily diet of raw fruits and salads, and sufficient proteins, and never eating to the point of fullness).

Exercise: For the next week, assess your hunger signals in relaxed somatic awareness before you eat. Notice whether the sensations in your stomach are genuine hunger, or stress, anxiety, depression, or other emotional-distress signals. If the sensations are not genuine hunger, go for a vigorous ten-to-twenty-minute walk outside while taking complete breaths before eating. Notice how you feel after the walk. Shift into relaxed somatic awareness before each meal and eat consciously in that state.

Prescription: Based on the above weeklong exercise and the insights you've gained from this evaluation, begin making conscious refinements in your diet guided by the clarity of somatic awareness. The feelings in your body and your stomach will tell you whether you need to eat smaller portions, eat or not eat snacks, or add or subtract certain foods in your diet. And trust that as you assess the following gateways and make healthy changes there, your dietary issues will naturally be resolved in the process.

The Breath Entrada *Checklist*

- Right now, in this moment, observe your breathing. Are you breathing through your nose or your mouth? Are you breathing into your abdomen or into your chest? Are these your regular breathing habits?
- Have you taken any complete breaths today?
- Are you sufficiently oxygenated right now? Are you "thirsting" for a breath? Do you feel mentally alert and energetic? Or mentally fuzzy and depleted?
- Stop right now and take three slow, deep, complete breaths.
- Do you breathe enough daily to oxygenate and energize your body fully?
- Are you a lazy breather, breathing just enough to "get by"?
- At least once a day, do you breathe consciously to revitalize and recharge your system?
- How many complete breaths do you take daily? (Or how many minutes of complete breathing do you do each day?)
- Do you take random full or complete breaths during the day?
- How often do you breathe fresh air in clean, natural environments?
- Based on your answers above, can you see any correlation

between your current breathing habits and your current energy and health levels or problems?

Assessment: Assess your current level of energy efficiency in your breathing habits on a scale of 1 to 10.

Prescription: Write a doable daily breathing prescription that will enhance your oxygen and energy intake. The last section of Chapter Five, "The Breath Gateway," has a variety of useful suggestions that you can use or adapt to your own situation and needs. But ideally you should incorporate one full session of complete breathing (five to ten minutes minimum) and random complete breaths during the day. The short-term purpose of this prescription is to begin sufficiently oxygenating your system on a daily basis. The long-term purpose is to train your body to breathe correctly and efficiently on its own. The results will be increased vitality and health, and a deeper somatic relationship to spirit energy through the breath.

The Water Entrada Checklist

- How many glasses of water do you drink a day on average?
- How many combined glasses of other beverages do you drink a day on average?
- Ideally, your water intake should triple your intake of other beverages. What is your current ratio of water to other beverages?
- Does your urine tend to be clear or light yellow, or does it tend toward a darker yellow?
- Notice the correlation between your answer to the question above and your answers to the first three questions preceding it. (The more water you drink, the lighter the color of your urine

will be, because the water is keeping your system clean. The less water you drink, the darker your urine will tend to be, because toxins are accumulating in your system.)

• How physically active are you on a daily basis? Include your work, home, and exercise habits. In light of the above answer, do you think you are sufficiently hydrating your body per amount of physical energy expended?

• How often do you work up a sweat?

• In the light of your answers to the above questions, can you see a correlation between your water intake and your current energy and health levels or problems?

Assessment: Based on your answers to these questions and in the light of the eight-glasses-per-day minimum, assess the degree to which you are meeting, or not meeting, your daily water needs. Rate the efficiency of your daily hydration on a scale of 1 to 10.

Prescription: Write out a daily water schedule for the coming week so that you meet the recommended eight glasses minimum per day. Beginning your day with a large glass of water is a good idea. (You can sip it slowly while you do your complete breathing exercise.) Drink periodically so that your body can absorb the water. Keep a large water bottle and glass nearby while you work. If it's practical, keep water in the glass at all times, and take random sips.

The Nature Entrada Checklist

• Do you take nature for granted in your life?
• How often—daily, weekly, monthly—do you go out in nature?
• How much time do you spend there?
• Do you notice a difference in how you feel after spending time in nature?

• Do the following brief exercise: Recall a time when you experienced the presence and power of nature. Then shift into somatic awareness and relive this moment right where you are. See it and feel it now as it was then. Do this for at least thirty seconds. Then open your eyes. Notice how you feel now compared to a minute ago. Notice how simply visualizing nature changes your state.

• Having done the above exercise, can you feel an instinctive desire in your body and mind to be in the presence of nature?

• Is there a serene nature environment conveniently located near you? Perhaps in your backyard? A small park in your neighborhood or an outdoor or indoor garden where you work?

• Are you taking advantage of the nature that is available to you?

• List all of the nature locations within thirty minutes of your house. Include local parks and gardens, mountain hiking trails, golf courses; your backyard; your neighborhood, if the houses have lots of trees and plants; or even an indoor garden in your house or where you work.

• Based on your answers to the above questions, can you see any correlation between your current level of contact with nature and your current energy and health levels or problems?

• Can you see how you might begin to incorporate nature more into your daily life and feel the positive effects that might have?

Assessment: On a scale of 1 to 10, intuitively assess your current level of nature contact and nature nourishment or undernourishment. Tune into your body in relaxed somatic awareness and it will tell you.

Prescription: Write a simple, doable nature prescription that will bring the healing presence and power of nature more into your life. Reread the suggestions given near the end of Chapter Nine, "The Nature Gateway." They will be useful here.

The Exercise **Entrada** *Checklist*

• How much do you exercise daily? Weekly? (Include activities like gardening, household chores, walking, climbing stairs, or any regular physical work or exertion.) Which of the following best describes you? (a) In excellent physical condition; (b) In good physical condition; (c) In average physical condition; (d) In poor physical condition.

• If you are in excellent physical condition, congratulations! If not, have you ever been? If so, how long has it been since you were in excellent shape? Do you remember how it felt to be in great shape?

• What do you think stands in the way of your getting into excellent condition? Write down every perceived obstacle between you and physical fitness.

• Close your eyes and imagine the following: See yourself walking briskly; see yourself dancing energetically; see yourself jogging; see yourself hiking a mountain trail; see yourself on a stair-climber at the gym; see yourself doing any other form of exercise that appeals to you, whether tennis, in-line skating, playing soccer, etc. Notice which activities feel the most exciting or rewarding to your body. Pay very close attention to the feelings—physical, emotional, and energetic—that each visualization stimulates in your body.

• Which one(s) "got your juices going" the most?

• Having done the above visualizations, can you feel your body's instinctive desire for vigorous or expressive movement and exercise?

• In the light of this, feel your body's current exercise needs. Is your body fulfilled in this area? Is it starved? Is it lethargic? What exactly do you feel?

• Do you believe you could get into excellent condition if you wanted to? If not, why not? If so, what would it take, and how long would it take?

• What form of exercise would you choose to do?

Assessment: On a scale of 1 to 10, intuitively assess your current fitness level. Again, on a scale of 1 to 10, assess the degree to which your body *feels satisfied* with the amount of exercise it is getting. (This is different than standard fitness. Tune into your body with somatic awareness for this one.) Can you feel any correlation between your current exercise status and your current energy and health levels or problems?

Prescription: In the light of your answers to the above questions, write a simple, doable, one-month exercise prescription. It's important to listen to your body and choose a form of exercise that it likes or can enjoy, rather than choose one that you (or anyone else) think is good for it. At the end of the month, make another assessment and write a follow-up prescription for an ongoing exercise program.

The Soul Entrada Checklist

• Do you tend to carry and accumulate stress and tension in your body without releasing them?

• How often do you feel pressured, restless, stressed, in a rush?

• How often do you feel calm, clear, focused, and purposeful?

• When was the last time you felt profound peace, relaxation, or connected to Spirit?

• What caused or allowed the experience?

• Do you think such spiritual experiences can happen only randomly or by chance?

• Close your eyes, relax into somatic awareness, and recall that spiritual experience. Feel, see, and remember it as vividly as possible. Do this for at least thirty seconds.

• Having done the above visualization, do you notice that you feel different than you did minutes ago? Can you feel that your state has changed?

• Having done this, can you feel your body and mind's instinctive desire for peace, deep relaxation, and spiritual connection, i.e., for positive "altered states"?

• Have you practiced some regular discipline, such as conscious relaxation, meditation, prayer, or yoga?

• If you do regularly engage in a somatic or meditative discipline, how well are you able to integrate that peace or calmness into your ordinary life? What other benefits do you notice?

• If you don't regularly engage in a somatic or meditative discipline, can you feel any correlation between this and your current levels of energy or stress, mental clarity, and overall health?

Assessment: On a scale of 1 to 10, in the light of your answers to the above questions, estimate your current level of relaxation, balance, peace, or spiritual connection. Again on a scale of 1 to 10, estimate your current level of *responsibility for developing* the above qualities in your life.

Prescription: Write a doable prescription for incorporating some somatic and meditative discipline into your daily life. If you already have, determine if you need to adapt or increase what you're already doing in order to bring more energy, clarity, calmness, and peace into your life.

The Relationship Entrada Checklist

- Do you enjoy being with others?
- Do you generally trust others?
- Do you feel cautious, uncertain, apprehensive, or mistrustful of others?
- How often—daily and/or weekly—do you have meaningful or enjoyable contact with others?
- Do you tend to avoid others?
- Do you prefer being alone?
- Do you genuinely enjoy solitude?
- Do you ever feel lonely?
- Do you have a good relationship with yourself? (Are you a kind and supportive friend to yourself?)
- Do you see any link between your relationship with yourself and your ability, or inability, to be in relationships with others?
- Are you currently involved in an intimate emotional and sexual relationship?
- If so, do you feel an open, trusting connection with that person?
- In this relationship, how much of yourself do you reveal, and how much of yourself do you hide?
- List the aspects of the relationship that give you energy and happiness, and rejuvenate you.
- List the aspects of the relationship that drain or deplete you, or are problematic or unresolved.
- What are your partner's negative qualities or liabilities in the relationship? What are yours? Do you see any connection between the two?
- In general, do your relationships with others give more energy than they take, or take more energy than they give?

• If you are not in a relationship, do you feel a longing to be in one?

• Do you judge yourself for not being in a relationship?

• To what degree do relationship issues occupy your attention?

• Can you see any correlation between the relationship issues in your life and your current energy and health levels or problems?

Assessment: On a scale of 1 to 10, how satisfied are you with your key life relationships? On a scale of 1 to 10, how satisfied are you with your relationship with yourself?

Prescription: In the light of your answers to the above questions, write down at least five specific things you can do to shift your relationships with others, and with yourself, into the realm of benign, healthy, intimate, and respectful human relations. This may include communicating more openly and truthfully with others, holding firmer boundaries with others, being more considerate, attentive, open, or expressive with others. Now, for each of these five things, write down a specific person or relationship in which you can practice this. In the next week, find a way to take one action in relation to another person for each of these five things. Make this an ongoing inquiry in your life and see what is revealed.

The Reciprocity Entrada *Checklist*

• When was the last time you went out of your way to help someone you knew for the sake of friendship?

• When was the last time you went out of your way to help a stranger out of altruism?

• Are you able to derive a sense of personal pleasure and meaning through helping or serving others?

• Do you regularly do some form of service or actions that benefit others?

• Do you believe that we're all in competition for insufficient resources, whether they be love, money, security, etc.?

• If you answered yes to the above question, can you feel any stress or anxiety associated with this belief? Can you feel how it subtly separates you from others?

• To what degree are you chronically preoccupied with your own survival and/or personal convenience or comfort?

• Do you feel there is an inherent conflict between taking care of your own needs and helping others?

• On a scale of 1 to 10, how high would you rate the importance of altruistic action for you, in your present life?

• How much of your life is focused on attending to the needs of others? Include children, employees, animals, etc.

• Recall a time when you experienced increased energy, joy, or meaning from contributing to others. Close your eyes and relive the event, see the person(s) you helped, their response, and feel now what you felt then. Having done this, do you think incorporating some consistent form of altruism in your life would have a significantly positive impact on your energy, your self-esteem, your relationship to others and to life?

• Can you see any correlation between your disposition and actions (or nonaction) in the area of reciprocity and your current energy and health levels, and in your sense of meaningful connection to others?

• How much energy is coming into your life through service?

• How much energy is being consumed in reluctant or imbalanced service, by taking on too much or doing things you really don't want to do?

Assessment: On a scale of 1 to 10, estimate your current level of altruism and reciprocity in life. To what degree are you being energized through altruistic action and operating in an altruistic spirit?

Prescription: In the light of your answers to the above questions, come up with a realistic plan for incorporating some form of altruistic service or behavior in your life. It could be performing "random acts of kindness" when you go out into the world. It could be donating time to a service-related organization. It could be making a concerted effort to discover needs of friends, family, or co-workers that you can help meet. It could be picking up at least one piece of litter from the street each day. If you are willing to look and act, you will be able to find a place to serve. The main thing is to access the Spirit of altruism and bring it more into your life.

Writing a Life Prescription

Now take all of the above prescriptions you've written and combine them into one complete, realistic, doable weekly schedule. Be creative. Adapt and combine if necessary. For example, you may not have time in your daily schedule to practice complete breathing, and meditate, and go out in nature, and exercise. But you can combine them, or mix and match. You can do complete breathing while meditating or hiking in nature, or while taking a brisk twenty-minute walk in your neighborhood, for example.

It is time to become your own primary physician and healer, to apply what you have learned (and perhaps already knew) about energy and health, to reach out and grasp the vitality and joy that are always available to you in abundant supply. Get out of your doctor's office and corner-store pharmacy, go within, and go out into nature and tap directly into Spirit's inexhaustible supply of energy.

EPILOGUE: A Sustainable Self:
Healing the Energy Crisis Within
by Connie Grauds, R.Ph.

We are in a crisis. In medicine we are in an economic crisis, but one that goes far beyond the problem of not being able to pay for medical care. We are in an environmental crisis, but it goes beyond the abuse and the neglect of our environment. Fundamentally, these are side effects of a greater crisis, and that is our failure to respect men, women, and children, a failure to honor humanity, to honor life, and a failure to ask with each thought, "Is this life-giving?" "Is this life sustaining?" "Or is this destructive?"

—Jeanne Achterberg, Ph.D., *Relationships Are the Best Medicine*

We heal in relationships. We are not separate. To quote shaman don Antonio, "There is only *one* disease—the disease of *dis*-connection." How we each manifest that disconnection is individual. Some people get ulcers, high blood pressure, or cancer. Some people lack good relationships or sufficient money. Some people suffer from anxiety, free-floating fears, or depression—the loss of a reason to live. To the shaman there is only one answer: Get connected. Facilitating connection to the life force is the shaman's way of healing a patient's ills.

Good relationships with those around us are vital to our health and well-being. In June of 1946, at the International Health Conference in New York, the preamble to the *Constitution of the World Health Organization* (WHO) defined health as "a state of complete physical, mental and social well-being and not merely the absence of disease or infirmity." This was formally adopted by conference representatives from sixty-one world states on April 7, 1948. This definition of health, which has not been amended since, is compatible with a shaman's definition of a sustainable self. We've had an international consensus on the holistic nature of health for over fifty years, yet we've been remiss in integrating its principles into our lives—or into our medical institutions.

When don Antonio visited the United States a few years ago, his first trip out of the jungle, he was startled to observe that Americans were, as a people, spiritually ill. He said that before his visit, he had often wondered why the Americans he met in the jungle, with all their fancy clothing and money, seemed so spiritually depleted. Now, he said, he understood: the busy-ness of busi-ness had depleted our souls. As don Antonio and I stood in Grand Central Station in New York City at the peak rush hour of 5:30 P.M., he saw a hectic, materialistic people under pressure, separated from nature, "like ants, more and more ants hurrying about."

Ecological Medicine:
The Medicine of Relationship

Simply stated, improving human health is inextricably linked to restoring ecological well-being. The interconnectedness of all life is a fundamental biological truth.

—**Kenny Ausubel,** *Ecological Medicine*

Ecology is the dynamic interplay (the homeodynamics) of the relationships among all of nature's systems—the animal, vegetable, and mineral kingdoms. We have the ecology within our own bodies, the ecology of our surroundings, and the ecology of the dynamic interplay between the two. As I define it, ecological medicine is the medicine of right relationship with every aspect of life.

If we look at where our modern medicine has come from and where it is going, we get an overview that looks something like this: Allopathic medicine, the basis of modern Western medicine, is based on a system of looking at body parts as separate from each other. If a patient is suffering from bronchitis, it is only the lungs that need to be considered. If a patient has thyroid cancer, such as I had, it was believed that only the thyroid gland was involved. Take my story to make a point. When my primary-care physician said the visible lump in my throat was from my thyroid gland, she ordered thyroid tests to be done. Intuitively realizing that perhaps there was more going on in my body than in just my thyroid gland, I insisted on a full panel of blood and electrolytes being done with a complete physical. My physician objected, saying all that wasn't necessary for a thyroid problem. I got my way in the end. I wasn't too surprised to hear from my physician the next morning at nine o'clock sharp. The tests revealed that, while my thyroid tests were normal, something was drastically wrong with my blood. I needed to see another specialist immediately. My intuition possibly saved my life. And the incident confirmed for me that I am not a skin bag full of disconnected parts, but a dynamic interdependent system, a whole human being.

Medicine began to realize some fifteen or twenty years ago that the mind and the body are connected. The terms *mind/body medicine* and *holistic medicine* were coined, reflecting the fact that our bodies are not separate systems but a whole, integrated system.

And medicine must treat and fully acknowledge the whole person.

Now medicine is taking the next step, expanding medicine beyond the body. Cutting-edge thinkers in modern medicine today are talking about "ecological medicine," healing within relationships outside of ourselves. Medicine is realizing the wisdom in the WHO's definition of health. Good relationships with family, friends, and our surroundings—society and nature—are as important to our healing as modern pharmaceuticals and surgery.

Interconnectedness is the only game in town when it comes to our health.

Environmental Medicine: Toxins Cause Diseases

The coming ecological disaster we worry about has already occurred, and goes on occurring. It takes place in the accounts of ourselves that separate ourselves from the world.

—James Hillman, *The Soul's Code*

Our environment is everything surrounding us: trees, birds, animals, land, oxygen, water, sun, sky, etc. If ecology is the dynamic interplay among these things (the "verb," so to speak) then the environment is the things themselves (the "noun," so to speak). Environmental medicine is the study of how the quality of the air, water, land, animals, plants, and everything around us affects our health. For example, medicine has known for some time now that there is a correlation among bad water, bad air, and bad health. The science of environmental medicine is now proving scientifically what we have intuitively known to be true.

Take cancer, for example. There is overwhelming evidence

that the increase in cancer rates we are experiencing is a direct result of avoidable and unavoidable exposure to carcinogens in the air, water, soil, and consumer products. We know that our industrialized society has dumped hundreds of industrial chemicals and carcinogens into our environment. As Dr. Samuel Epstein has noted, ". . . cancer is the only major adverse impact for which we can clearly relate a direct causal relationship between avoidable carcinogenic exposures and escalating trends. Cancer is thus a quantifiable manifestation of runaway industrial technologies that affect all of us." Not only are the fish, birds, and animals suffering because of it, but so are we humans. This is nothing new.

What is a new realization to most of us is that pharmaceutical drugs are also now fast becoming part of our environmental toxins. To paraphrase Andrew Weil, M.D., "If you want to find new drugs, you look to poisons, because there's no difference between a drug and a poison except dose. The word 'pharmacology' means the study of poisons. 'Toxicology' comes from the Greek word for bow (as in bow and arrow): *taxos*. Many poisons become useful drugs if you can lower the dose enough. All drugs become poisons if you push the dose high enough."

Some 50 to 95 percent of pharmaceutical drugs are excreted from the body chemically unchanged. Consequently, huge quantities of potentially poisonous pharmaceutical antibiotics, high-blood-pressure medication, oral contraceptives, radiopharmaceuticals, tranquilizers, painkillers, and chemotherapy medications are coming out of our urine or feces and going into our environment, with negative impacts on the ecosystems. It is alarming (in fact, *susto* inducing) to know that the very drug we take in hopes of healing us as individuals may in fact be doing more harm to us as a species and to all the species that live on Earth with us.

"Do no harm" is a physician's Hippocratic oath. Yet our medicine today seems to do just that.

Many of the toxins we're talking about here are synthetic in nature, made by man. As we look to our relationship with nature, consider the following enlightening statistic from *The Lost Language of Plants,* by Stephen Buhner. He writes, "In people, increases in cancers exactly parallel the decrease of diverse plants as foods and medicines. Complex plant combinations keep disease conditions in check in people, just as they do in pigeons and in ecosystems." If we could stop the synthetic overload of toxins and start feasting on, and basking in, Mother Nature's cornucopia of flora and foodstuffs, we would experience the reality of the basic shamanic principle that "nature heals."

Sustainable Medicine, Sacred Sustainability

Where does the environment stop and I begin, and can I begin at all without being in some place, deeply involved in, nurtured by the nature of the world?

—James Hillman, *The Soul's Code*

How can we call a medicine a medicine when it can be potentially toxic to us in the long run? I daresay that our synthetic pharmaceuticals might not be the ultimate medicine by this definition. While synthetic pharmaceuticals have indeed saved my life and the lives of countless others, perhaps there are natural alternatives that might have done the job.

Let's look at our natural medicines—our plant medicines, for example. Sara Warber, M.D., and her colleagues have written that "with the increasing demand for plant products as medicine, we need a set of principles to guide our actions. Medical ethics, which until now have focused on human concerns, must expand to include notions about the relationship of humans and plants." They go on to report that among the native peoples of the Great Lakes areas, teachers of herbal knowledge have sacred principles by which they gather plants. These gathering principles focus on respect, purpose, stewardship, and regeneration—all part of what I would term sacred sustainability.

I believe that for a plant medicine to be truly a medicine, it should be a medicine that is completely part of a whole and healthy energy cycle as well as a medicine that is ecologically sound. It should be a medicine that includes organic farming practices, but is beyond organic; a medicine that is part of fair trade practices, but goes beyond fair trade; a medicine that is ecologically and ethically sound—a medicine of "right relationship."

Shamans are experts at working with nature to grow ecologically sound plant medicines in order to have sustainable medicines. Shamans believe plants to be spirit beings. So they also pray over the plant medicines as they sow them, harvest them, and before they give them out as medicines. Sustainable medicine combines both the ancient shamanic principle and the modern ecological concept of "right relationship"; right relationship to the Earth, to the plants themselves, to the farmers and shamans who grow them, with ethical marketing, and with the people who take them. If all these relationships are truly "right," they form a complete and healthy energy cycle. If we pray over them, with them, and for them, they become a sacred sustainable medicine. As a pharmacist, as a natural-medicine expert, and as a shaman, I would call that the ultimate sustainable medicine.

Eco-Therapy: The Shaman's Medicine

A shaman's mysterious healing practices are a blend of medicine and spirit. The rain forest shamans have an intimate relationship with the healing spirits of nature. They summon these healing energies and transfer this energy to their patients during the healing.

—**Connie Grauds,** *Jungle Medicine*

We can connect to the life force ourselves, no shaman needed. We can manage our own "eco-therapy," a term I have coined to mean healing in relationship to our environment. Eco-therapy heals by enhancing the homeodynamic balance of the ecology inside and outside ourselves.

Nature, when it's wild and vital, lives in ecstasy. We can tap into an inexhaustible supply of ecstatic energy by plugging into nature to the fullest—by wrapping ourselves in the arms of Mother Nature herself and feeding on the breast of the energetic life force. With his eyes twinkling with the light of Spirit like two great beaming flashlights, don Antonio, for me the embodiment of a sustainable self, once looked at me and said, "Why do you think I live in the jungle?" What a simple, yet profound, teaching.

This book is an introductory course on eco-therapy. I teach an extensive experiential program to train people to become shamanic eco-therapists, to become healers. In this course, we spend as much time outdoors as possible, learning nature's secrets directly, in relationship. In the exotic jungles, vast rain forests, and rich wildernesses around the globe, the healing secrets of nature reveal themselves to whoever will receive them. We learn to tap into deep sources of energy that revitalize and propel our life's purpose forward.

In this course, we accept sustainability as the new standard: sustainability of the self (energy and radiant health) and sustainability of our medicines (right relationship, nontoxic medicines). We know that sustaining the self is becoming increasingly difficult, and that lack of energy is the number-one complaint in physicians' offices today. We learn that science shows us that there are lifestyle habits that deplete personal energy. Shamans are known experts at the techniques of harnessing the powers of nature to respirit and energize our lives, to achieve the sustainable self. We learn to create our own Garden of Eden around us. Ultimately, we learn the secret behind don Antonio's statement about living in the jungle—the Garden of Eden we call the rain forest.

With this book, you can do basic eco-therapy for yourself—heal yourself—in your own backyard. Eco-therapy is about tapping into the inexhaustible, ubiquitous spirit of nature and life itself, to energize and to heal—the shaman's medicine. It's about learning to set up a dynamic relationship, or personal ecology, between our individual spirit and the Great Spirit that surrounds us, completing the ultimate energy circuit. You now know how to do this for yourself. You have learned the secrets of a sustainable self.

Once we are well in our bodies and souls, we will have enough energy to share with life around us, to give back. When we are lacking, we are naturally "self-absorbed." We care only about getting our needs met. As we are nourished enough and filled up with the energy of life, we begin to have desires to give thanks to the resources that gave us our life back. Out of gratitude, we begin to give thanks for the spirited medicine that has made us well and whole. From thankfulness, caring and passion grow. We begin naturally to care for Mother Earth, the welfare of her life-giving water and her breath of life we call air. We feel closer, more connected, to those that inhabit this planet with us, the animals and the plants around us, and our community. The feeling of fear that accompanies our earlier disconnect is leaving us. We connect more fully with the spirit of life as each day goes on. We realize that life has meaning, everything has meaning, and that our own personal lives have spiritual meaning, too. Our soul is beginning to heal. Thanks to this spirited medicine, our soul has come to life.

Thank you, Spirit!

REFERENCES

Anaya, Rudolfo. *Jalamanta*. Warner, 1997.

Atmanspacher, H; Römer, H; Walach, H. Weak quantum theory: complementarity and entanglement in physics and beyond. *Foundations of Physics*. 2002.

Ausubel, Kenny. *Ecological Medicine*. Sierra Club Books, 2004.

Barbour, Ian. *When Science Meets Religion*. HarperSanFrancisco, 2000.

Bratman, S. *St. John's Wort and Depression*. Prima Health, 1999.

Braud, W. Wellness implications of retroactive intentional influence: exploring an outrageous hypothesis. *Alternative Therapies in Health & Medicine*. 2000.

Brooks, M. The weirdest link: quantum entanglement. *New Scientist*. 27 March 2004.

———Vive la weirdness! Editorial on quantum entanglement; p.3.

Buhner, Stephen. *The Lost Language of Plants*. Chelsea Green Publishing, 2002.

Chalmers, D.J. The puzzle of conscious experience. *Scientific American*. 1995.

Clarke, C.J.S. The nonlocality of mind. *Journal of Consciousness Studies*. 1995.

Darling, David. *Soul Search*. Villard Books, 1995. Quotation from: First world. *Omni*. Winter 1995.

Dossey, Larry. *Reinventing Medicine*. HarperSanFrancisco, 1999.

Dossey, Larry. The case for nonlocality. *Reinventing Medicine*. HarperSanFrancisco, 1999: 37–84.

Dossey, Larry. *Recovering the Soul*. Bantam Books, 1989.

Dossey, Larry. Emerging theories: The return of prayer. *Alternative Therapies in Health and Medicine*. 1997; 3(6):10–17, 133–120.

Dossey, Larry. Living dangerously: risk-taking and health. *Alternative Therapies in Health and Medicine.* 2003; 9(6): 10–14, 94–96.

Dossey, Larry. Black Monday syndrome: When dread means dead. *Meaning & Medicine.* Bantam Books, 1991.

Eccles, J.C. *Evolution of the Brain, Creation of the Self.* Routledge, 1991.

Epstein, Samuel. *The Politics of Cancer Revisited.* East Ridge Press, 1998.

Giberson, Karl; Yerxa, Donald. *Species of Origins: America's Search for a Creation Story.* Rowman & Littlefield, 2002.

Grauds, Connie. *Jungle Medicine.* The Center for Spirited Medicine, 2004.

Grauds, C. *Kava and Anxiety.* Prima Health, 1999.

Hillman, James. *The Soul's Code.* Warner Books, 1996.

Karasek, R.L.; Theorell, T.; Schwartz, J.E.; Schnall, P.L.; Pieper, C.F.; Michela, J.L. Job characteristics in relation to the prevalence of myocardial infarction. *American Journal of Public Health.* 1988.

Keyes, Ralph. *Chancing It: Why We Take Risks.* Little, Brown and Company, 1985.

Nadeau, Robert; Kafatos, Menas. *The Non-Local Universe: The New Physics and Matters of the Mind.* Oxford University Press, 1999.

Olshansky, B; Dossey, L. Retroactive prayer: A preposterous hypothesis? *British Medical Journal.* December 20, 2000.

Rachman, S. *Fear and Courage.* W.H. Freeman, 1978.

Radin, Dean. *The Conscious Universe.* HarperSanFrancisco, 1997.

Shields, J.W. *Lymph, lymph glands, and homeostasis.* Lymphology, v25, n4, December 1992.

Starfield, B. Is US health really the best in the world? *Journal of the American Medical Association.* July 26, 2000.

Wald, G. *Bulletin of the Foundation for Mind-Being Research.* September 1988.

Warber, Sara, et al. Environmental Ethics: Finding a Moral Compass for Human-Plant Interaction. *Alternative Therapies.* March/April 2003. v9.

Watson, Peter. *War on the Mind: The Military Uses and Abuses of Psychology.* Basic Books, 1978.

Work in America: Report of a Special Task Force to the Secretary of Health, Education, and Welfare. Cambridge, MA: MIT Press, 1973.

INDEX

ABOUT THE AUTHORS

Constance Grauds, R.Ph., is an assistant professor of clinical pharmacy, University of California at San Francisco. A nationally known lecturer on natural medicine and indigenous healing practices, Grauds is the only experienced pharmacist to have undergone a decade of shamanic training in the Amazon. She is president of the Association of Natural Medicine Pharmacists, which provides education on natural medicine to thousands of health-care professionals nationwide; director of the Center for Spirited Medicine; and the author of *Kava and Anxiety* and *Jungle Medicine*.

Doug Childers is a freelance book doctor, ghostwriter, editor, writing coach, and novelist. He has published on East-West spirituality, psychology, shamanism, political history, and mind-body health. He co-authored the critically acclaimed memoir *The White-Haired Girl,* and *Divine Interventions*, a nonfiction work on the miraculous. He lives in San Rafael, California, and can be contacted at dougchilders@comcast.net.